D1323707

Evidence-Based Psychiatry

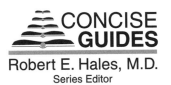

CONCISE
GUIDES

Robert E. Hales, M.D.
Series Editor

CONCISE GUIDE TO
Evidence-Based Psychiatry

Gregory E. Gray, M.D., Ph.D.

Professor and Chairman
Department of Psychiatry and Human Behavior
Charles R. Drew University of Medicine and Science
Los Angeles, California

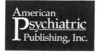

American
Psychiatric
Publishing, Inc.

Washington, DC
London, England

Copyright © 2004 American Psychiatric Publishing, Inc.
ALL RIGHTS RESERVED

Typeset in Adobe's Times and Helvetica

Manufactured in the United States of America on acid-free paper
07   06   05   04   03   5   4   3   2   1
First Edition

American Psychiatric Publishing, Inc.
1000 Wilson Boulevard
Arlington, VA 22209-3901
www.appi.org

Library of Congress Cataloging-in-Publication Data
Gray, Gregory E., 1954-
    Concise guide to evidence-based psychiatry / Gregory E. Gray.—1st ed.
        p. ; cm. — (Concise guides)
    Includes bibliographical references and index.
    ISBN 1-58562-096-3 (alk. paper)
    1. Evidence-based psychiatry. I. Title: Evidence-based psychiatry. II. Title. III. Concise guides (American Psychiatric Publishing)
    [DNLM: 1. Evidence-Based Medicine—methods. 2. Psychiatry. WM 100 G779c 2003]
    RC455.2.E94G73 2003
    616.89—dc21   2003052160

British Library Cataloguing in Publication Data
A CIP record is available from the British Library.

CONTENTS

LIST OF TABLES

6 Systematic Reviews and Meta-Analyses

7 Clinical Practice Guidelines

8 Diagnostic Tests

9 Surveys of Disease Frequency

10 Studies of Risk or Harm

11 Studies of Prognosis

12 Evaluating Your Performance

13 Learning and Practicing Evidence-Based Psychiatry

14 Teaching Evidence-Based Medicine to Psychiatry Residents

Appendix A: Glossary

Appendix B: Statistical Formulas and Tables

LIST OF FIGURES

6 Systematic Reviews and Meta-Analyses

8 Diagnostic Tests

11 Studies of Prognosis

INTRODUCTION

to the Concise Guides Series

The Concise Guides Series from American Psychiatric Publishing, Inc., provides, in an accessible format, practical information for psychiatrists, psychiatry residents, and medical students working in a variety of treatment settings, such as inpatient psychiatry units, outpatient clinics, consultation-liaison services, and private office settings. The Concise Guides are meant to complement the more detailed information found in lengthier psychiatry texts.

The Concise Guides address topics of special concern to psychiatrists in clinical practice. The books in this series contain a detailed table of contents, along with an index, tables, figures, and other charts for easy access. The books are designed to fit into a lab coat pocket or jacket pocket, which makes them a convenient source of information. References have been limited to those most relevant to the material presented.

Robert E. Hales, M.D., M.B.A.
Series Editor, Concise Guides

PREFACE

It is almost impossible these days to attend a conference or to pick up a journal and not come across the phrase "evidence-based." Despite this increased emphasis on evidence-based practice, most psychiatrists and other mental health professionals remain unfamiliar with the methods and philosophy of evidence-based medicine (EBM).

This Concise Guide was written with three audiences in mind. The first audience consists of psychiatry residency program directors and faculty who are looking for a brief introduction to EBM. Now that the Accreditation Council for Graduate Medical Education requires that all residents develop EBM skills as part of the "practice-based learning and improvement" core competency, there is a need for psychiatry faculty to become familiar with EBM in order to incorporate the teaching of EBM skills into residency programs. This Concise Guide can serve as an introduction to EBM, and Chapter 14 includes suggestions for teaching EBM in psychiatry residency programs.

The second audience is psychiatry residents and other mental health trainees. Several textbooks on the topic of EBM are available, but most of them are oriented toward residents in primary care specialties, not in psychiatry. This Concise Guide focuses on the needs of psychiatry residents and of other mental health trainees by emphasizing the information resources of most use in finding answers to clinical questions in psychiatric practice. In addition, examples are drawn from the psychiatric literature, rather than from general medicine or surgery.

The third audience consists of psychiatrists and other mental health professionals who wish to learn about EBM on their own and to incorporate EBM into their daily practice. This Concise Guide can be used both as an introduction to the topic and a ready reference for searching the literature and appraising evidence.

This Concise Guide cannot cover the entire field of EBM and clinical epidemiology in depth. For individuals seeking further information, references are given in the text and suggested Web sites are listed in tables. In addition, suggestions for further study are given in Chapter 13.

The author has found learning and practicing EBM to be both stimulating and enjoyable and hopes that readers of this Concise Guide will, too.

INTRODUCTION TO EVIDENCE-BASED MEDICINE

The phrase "evidence-based" is appearing with increasing frequency in the psychiatric literature, and the 2001 volume of the journal *Psychiatric Services* was dedicated to evidence-based psychiatry (Talbott 2001); a collection of the articles is also available in book form (American Psychiatric Association 2003). Despite the increasing use of this term, even leaders of American psychiatry often appear unfamiliar with the methods and philosophy of evidence-based medicine (EBM), frequently equating it with cost-cutting practice guidelines or with "cookbook medicine" (Borenstein 2001). What, then, is evidence-based medicine, and how did it come about?

■ CLINICAL PRACTICE IS NOT ALWAYS EVIDENCE BASED

Over the past few years, evidence has accumulated to suggest that there is a significant gap between the knowledge obtained from clinical trials regarding effective treatments for mental disorders and the actual treatment of patients in clinical practice (Drake et al. 2001; Lehman and Steinwachs 1998; U.S. Department of Health and Human Services 1999; Young et al. 2001). Similar discrepancies have been noted in other fields of medicine, where practice often lags years behind research findings (Egger et al. 2001; Geyman 2000; Haines and Donald 1998; Haines and Jones 1994).

There are also wide variations in the way psychiatry and other medical specialties are practiced (Geddes and Harrison 1997; Geyman 2000). Clearly, some methods of treatment must be more effective than others and have more research to support their use, yet surveys conducted in academic medical centers have found that up to 40% of clinical decisions are unsupported by evidence from the research literature (Geddes et al. 1996; Greenhalgh 2001).

Two general types of information problems contribute to patients receiving less than optimal care (Gray 2002; Haynes et al. 1997). The first problem is one of "information overload," which creates difficulties for clinicians who want to determine which treatments are truly most effective. There are thousands of medical journals and millions of articles; therefore, no psychiatrist or other clinician should expect to keep up with all of the developments in his or her field. Furthermore, when one looks at the results of various studies, they often appear to be contradictory. In part, this is caused by false-positive and false-negative results, which often arise from small studies (Collins and MacMahon 2001; also see Chapter 5). One could consult review articles to summarize the literature, but most such reviews are "journalistic" or "narrative" reviews, not systematic reviews (see Chapter 6). As a result, such articles are subject to the biases of the review's author(s), both in terms of studies cited and in the method of summarizing conflicting results (Cook et al. 1998; Egger et al. 2001; Greenhalgh 2001). Textbook chapters have the added problem of being out of date (Sackett et al. 2000). All of this contributes to the lag before advances in treatment are recognized and find their way into practice.

The second type of information problem causes ineffective treatments to be adopted or maintained. Here the problem is not a lack of information, but rather the uncritical acceptance of available information. This may occur for a variety of reasons, such as over-reliance on one's own clinical experiences or on expert opinion, the uncritical acceptance of results of single studies, and the excessive influence of pharmaceutical companies through advertising and sponsorship of speakers (Greenhalgh 2001; Sackett et al. 2000).

A variety of approaches have been suggested to close the gap between research and practice, thus improving the quality of patient care (Grol 2001; Haines and Donald 2002; National Health Service [NHS] Centre for Reviews and Dissemination 1999; Oxman et al. 1995). One such approach is EBM.

■ PHILOSOPHY OF EVIDENCE-BASED MEDICINE

EBM has been described as "partly a philosophy, partly a skill, and partly the application of a set of tools" (Dawes 1999, p. ix). David Sackett, often considered the father of EBM, has defined it as "the conscientious, explicit, and judicious use of current best evidence in making decisions about the care of individual patients" (Sackett et al. 1996, p. 71). It is the application of "a knowledge of medical informatics and clinical epidemiology to the treatment of individual patients" (Gray 2002, p. 5) and involves "the integration of best research evidence with clinical expertise and patient values" (Sackett et al. 2000, p. 1).

Contrary to the assertions of some critics that EBM devalues clinical judgment and the "art" of medicine (Borenstein 2001; Rushton 2001; Williams and Garner 2002), clinical expertise continues to play an important role in EBM by allowing the clinician to integrate research evidence, patient preferences, and clinical state in making decisions about patient care (Guyatt et al. 2000; Haynes et al. 2002a, 2000b; Straus and McAlister 2000). Rather than being "cookbook medicine," EBM actually empowers clinicians to make their own decisions about patient care, guided by the best available evidence to support those decisions (Gray 2002; Lipman 2000; Trinder 2000a). Finally, EBM places great emphasis on patient preferences and values and encourages patient-centered care (Guyatt et al. 2000; Hope 2002).

■ DEVELOPMENT OF EVIDENCE-BASED MEDICINE AND PSYCHIATRY

EBM had its origin in the Department of Clinical Epidemiology and Biostatistics at McMaster University in Canada (Guyatt 2002). In

1981, members of that department began publishing a series of articles in the *Canadian Medical Association Journal* that were intended to teach clinicians how to critically appraise the medical literature. In 1990, they began to move beyond teaching critical appraisal skills and developing a new philosophy of medical education, which they termed "evidence-based medicine." In this new model, physicians would rely heavily on the medical research literature, rather than on textbooks or tradition, when approaching patient care problems. This new approach to medical education was described in some detail in an article that appeared in the *Journal of the American Medical Association* (*JAMA*) in 1992 (Evidence-Based Medicine Working Group 1992). At about the same time, the group at McMaster was asked to update the articles that had appeared in the *Canadian Medical Association Journal,* as the basis for a series of articles that would appear in *JAMA.* The Evidence-Based Medicine Working Group, consisting of several members of the McMaster faculty, as well as several American academic physicians, was formed to accomplish this task. The group went on to publish a series of 25 articles that appeared in *JAMA* between 1993 and 2000. These articles have recently been revised and published in book form (Guyatt and Rennie 2002); they are also available, in their original form, at the Centre for Health Evidence Web site (http://www.cche.net/usersguides/main.asp).

Although EBM was developed in Canada and described in *JAMA,* it has probably had its greatest impact in Britain. In part, this was because of the support of the National Health Service (Baker and Kleijnen 2000; Ferguson and Russell 2000; Reynolds 2000; Trinder 2000c). The NHS viewed EBM as a way to both improve the quality of care and to control costs by identifying and promoting therapies that worked and by eliminating therapies that were ineffective or harmful. The NHS funds university-based centers for EBM, surgery, child health, general practice, pathology, pharmacotherapy, nursing, dentistry, and mental health, as well as the NHS Centre for Reviews and Dissemination and the United Kingdom's Cochrane Centre (Baker and Kleijnen 2000; Sackett et al. 1996). In addition, the BMJ Publishing Group publishes several evidence-based journals and the semiannual publication *Clinical Evidence*, which is distributed to general practitioners by the NHS (Baker and Kleijnen 2000; Barton 2001). The evidence-based practice philosophy in the United Kingdom has expanded beyond medicine and health care to include social work, education, probation, and public policy (Davies and Boruch 2001; Hammersley 2000; Thyer 2002; Trinder 2000b, 2000c).

Given the influence of managed care on American medicine, one might have expected EBM to have had an equally large impact in the United States; however, this has not been the case. Perhaps the reason is that for-profit health maintenance organizations have focused on controlling cost, rather than improving quality, and therefore have not actively promoted EBM. Although the Federal Agency for Healthcare Research and Quality (AHRQ) has funded a series of evidence-based practice centers that produce systematic reviews (AHRQ 2003), it too has played a relatively minor role in promoting the teaching and practice of EBM. Instead, the dissemination of EBM in the United States has largely been the result of professional organizations, such as the American College of Physicians, and journals, such as *JAMA, ACP Journal Club,* and the *Journal of the American Board of Family Practice* (Geyman 2000; Gray 2002; Guyatt 2002). As a result, most instruction about EBM occurs in primary care departments, with several medical schools (e.g., Duke, Yale, the University of California at San Francisco, and the University of Washington) having faculty active in this field. This will change with the adoption of the new general competencies for residency programs that require that all residents become familiar with the methods of EBM (Accreditation Council for Graduate Medical Education 2001).

Although the first article on "evidence-based psychiatry" appeared in 1995 (Bilsker and Goldner 1995), EBM has had less of an impact on psychiatry and other mental health disciplines than it has had on most medical specialties (Geddes 2000; Goss and Rowland 2000); however, there are indications that this is beginning to change (Geddes and Carney 2001; Milne et al. 2000). In part, this resistance may be the result of a misunderstanding of EBM by many mental health professionals and the belief that their patients' individuality and the nonquantifiable aspects of psychotherapy preclude the application of EBM to psychotherapeutic interventions (Geddes 2000; Geddes et al. 1997; Goss and Rowland 2000; Mace et al. 2001; Parry 2000).

As in other specialties, the influence of EBM on psychiatry has been greatest in the United Kingdom, again because of the role of the NHS, as well as the efforts of the Centre for Evidence-Based Mental Health at the University of Oxford (Baker and Kleijnen 2000; Ferguson and Russell 2000; Geddes 2000). These efforts have been aided by the journal *Evidence-Based Mental Health,* which is published jointly by the BMJ Publishing Group, the Royal College of Psychiatrists, and the British Psychological Society (Geddes et al. 1997). In addition, skill in applying EBM is tested in the critical appraisal paper that is now included in part II of the membership exam of the Royal College of Psychiatrists (Dhar 2001; Geddes 2000).

In the United States, there has been support for the evidence-based mental health practices of the AHRQ and the Robert Wood Johnson Foundation (Torrey et al. 2001). In addition, the 2001 volume of *Psychiatric Services* was dedicated to evidence-based psychiatry (Talbott 2001). However, much of the effort of these organizations has been directed toward the use of clinical practice guidelines, rather than to the teaching of EBM. At present, only 36% of U.S. psychiatry residency programs have specific instruction in EBM, and only one-half of these programs seem to have a reasonably comprehensive course of instruction (G. E. Gray, unpublished data, January 2002). This should change, however, with the adoption of the new general competencies for residency programs (Accreditation Council for Graduate Medical Education 2001), which will require competence in the methods of EBM.

■ REFERENCES

Accreditation Council for Graduate Medical Education: General competencies [ACGME Outcome Project Web site]. 2001. Available at: http://www.acgme.org/outcome/comp/compfull.asp. Accessed June 27, 2003

Agency for Healthcare Research and Quality: Evidence-based practice centers [AHRQ Web site]. March 2003. Available at: http://www.ahcpr.gov/clinic/epc/. Accessed June 27, 2003

American Psychiatric Association: Evidence-Based Practices in Mental Health Care. Washington, DC, American Psychiatric Association, 2003

Baker M, Kleijnen J: The drive towards evidence-based health care, in Evidence-Based Counseling and Psychological Therapies: Research and Applications. Edited by Rowland N, Goss S. Philadelphia, PA, Routledge, 2000, pp 13–29

Barton S: Using clinical evidence. BMJ 322:503–504, 2001

Bilsker D, Goldner EM: Evidence-based psychiatry. Can J Psychiatry 40:97–101, 1995

Borenstein D: Evidence-based psychiatry. Psychiatr News 36:3, 2001

Collins R, MacMahon S: Reliable assessment of the effects of treatment on mortality and major morbidity, I: clinical trials. Lancet 357:373–380, 2001

Cook DJ, Mulrow CD, Haynes RB: Synthesis of best evidence for clinical decisions, in Systematic Reviews: Synthesis of Best Evidence for Health Care Decisions. Edited by Mulrow C, Cook D. Philadelphia, PA, American College of Physicians, 1998, pp 5–12

Davies P, Boruch R: The Campbell Collaboration. BMJ 323:294–295, 2001

Dawes M: Preface, in Evidence-Based Practice: A Primer for Health Professionals. Edited by Dawes M, Davies P, Gray A, et al. New York, Churchill Livingstone, 1999, pp ix–x

Dhar R: Evidence-based journal clubs and the critical review paper. Psychiatr Bull 25:67–68, 2001

Drake RE, Goldman HH, Leff HS, et al: Implementing evidence-based practices in routine mental health settings. Psychiatr Serv 52:179–182, 2001

Egger M, Smith GD, O'Rourke K: Rationale, potentials, and promise of systematic reviews, in Systematic Reviews in Health Care. Edited by Egger M, Smith GD, Altman DG. London, BMJ Books, 2001, pp 3–19

Evidence-Based Medicine Working Group: Evidence-based medicine: a new approach to the teaching of medicine. JAMA 268:2420–2425, 1992

Ferguson B, Russell I: Towards evidence-based health care, in Evidence-Based Counseling and Psychological Therapies: Research and Applications. Edited by Rowland N, Goss S. Philadelphia, PA, Routledge, 2000, pp 30–43

Geddes J: Evidence-based practice in mental health, in Evidence-Based Practice: A Critical Appraisal. Edited by Trinder L, Reynolds S. Oxford, UK, Blackwell Scientific, 2000, pp 66–88

Geddes J, Carney S: Recent advances in evidence-based psychiatry. Can J Psychiatry 46:403–406, 2001

Geddes JR, Harrison PJ: Closing the gap between research and practice. Br J Psychiatry 171:220–225, 1997

Geddes JR, Game D, Jenkins NE, et al: What proportion of primary psychiatric interventions are based on evidence from randomised controlled trials? Qual Health Care 5:215–217, 1996

Geddes J, Reynolds S, Streiner D, et al: Evidence based practice in mental health. BMJ 315:1483–1484, 1997

Geyman JP: Evidence-based medicine in primary care: an overview, in Evidence-Based Clinical Practice: Concepts and Approaches. Edited by Geyman JP, Deyo RA, Ramsey SD. Boston, MA, Butterworth-Heinemann, 2000, pp 1–12

Goss S, Rowland N: Getting evidence into practice, in Evidence-Based Counseling and Psychological Therapies: Research and Applications. Edited by Rowland N, Goss S. Philadelphia, PA, Routledge, 2000, pp 191–205

Gray GE: Evidence-based medicine: an introduction for psychiatrists. J Psychiatr Pract 8:5–13, 2002

Greenhalgh T: How to Read a Paper: The Basics of Evidence Based Medicine, 2nd Edition. London, BMJ Books, 2001

Grol R: Improving the quality of medical care: building bridges among professional pride, payer profit, and patient satisfaction. JAMA 286:2578–2585, 2001

Guyatt G: Preface, in Users' Guides to the Medical Literature: A Manual for Evidence-Based Clinical Practice. Edited by Guyatt G, Rennie D. Chicago, IL, AMA Press, 2002, pp xiii–xvi

Guyatt G, Rennie D (eds); Users' Guides to the Medical Literature: A Manual for Evidence-Based Clinical Practice. Chicago, IL, AMA Press, 2002

Guyatt GH, Haynes RB, Jaeschke RZ, et al: Users' guides to the medical literature, XXV. Evidence-based medicine: principles for applying the users' guides to patient care. JAMA 284:1290–1296, 2000

Haines A, Donald A: Making better use of research findings. BMJ 317:72–75, 1998

Haines A, Donald A (eds): Getting Research Findings into Practice, 2nd Edition. London, BMJ Books, 2002

Haines A, Jones R: Implementing findings of research. BMJ 308:1488–1492, 1994

Hammersley M: Evidence-based practice in education and the contribution of educational research, in Evidence-Based Practice: A Critical Appraisal. Edited by Trinder L, Reynolds S. Oxford, UK, Blackwell Scientific, 2000, pp 163–184

Haynes RB, Sackett DL, Gray JA, et al: Transferring evidence from research into practice, II: getting the evidence straight. ACP J Club 126:A14–A16, 1997

Haynes RB, Devereaux PJ, Guyatt GH: Clinical expertise in the era of evidence-based medicine and patient choice. ACP J Club 136:A11–A14, 2002a

Haynes RB, Devereaux PJ, Guyatt GH: Physicians' and patients' choices in evidence based practice. BMJ 324:1350, 2002b

Hope T: Evidence-based patient choice and psychiatry. Evid Based Ment Health 5:100–101, 2002

Lehman AF, Steinwachs DM: Patterns of usual care for schizophrenia: initial results from the Schizophrenia Patient Outcomes Research Team (PORT) client survey. Schizophr Bull 24:11–20, 1998

Lipman T: Evidence-based practice in general practice and primary care, in Evidence-Based Practice: A Critical Appraisal. Edited by Trinder L, Reynolds S. Oxford, UK, Blackwell Scientific, 2000, pp 35–65

Mace C, Moorey S, Roberts B (eds): Evidence in the Psychological Therapies: A Critical Guide for Practitioners. Philadelphia, PA, Brunner-Routledge, 2001

Milne D, Keegan D, Paxton R, et al: Is the practice of psychological therapists evidence-based? Int J Health Care Qual Assur 13:8–14, 2000

National Health Service Centre for Reviews and Dissemination: Getting evidence into practice. Eff Health Care 5(1):1–16, 1999

Oxman AD, Thomson MA, Davis DA, et al: No magic bullet: a systematic review of 102 trials of interventions to improve professional practice. CMAJ 153:1423–1431, 1995

Parry G: Evidence-based psychotherapy: an overview, in Evidence-Based Counseling and Psychological Therapies: Research and Applications. Edited by Rowland N, Goss S. Philadelphia, PA, Routledge, 2000, pp 57–75

Reynolds S: The anatomy of evidence-based practice: principles and methods, in Evidence-Based Practice: A Critical Appraisal. Edited by Trinder L, Reynolds S. Oxford, UK, Blackwell Scientific, 2000, pp 17–34

Rushton JL: The burden of evidence. BMJ 323:349, 2001

Sackett DL, Rosenberg WMC, Gray JAM, et al: Evidence-based medicine: what it is and what it isn't. BMJ 312:71–72, 1996

Sackett DL, Strauss SE, Richardson WS, et al: Evidence-Based Medicine: How to Practice and Teach EBM, 2nd Edition. New York, Churchill Livingstone, 2000

Straus SE, McAlister FA: Evidence-based medicine: a commentary on common criticisms. CMAJ 163:837–841, 2000

Talbott JA: Business as usual: no way to enter 2001. Psychiatr Serv 52:7, 2001

Thyer BA: Evidence-based practice and clinical social work. Evid Based Ment Health 5:6–7, 2002

Torrey WC, Drake RE, Dixon L, et al: Implementing evidence-based practices for persons with severe mental illnesses. Psychiatr Serv 52:45–50, 2001

Trinder L: A critical appraisal of evidence-based practice, in Evidence-Based Practice: A Critical Appraisal. Edited by Trinder L, Reynolds S. Oxford, UK, Blackwell Scientific, 2000a, pp 212–241

Trinder L: Evidence-based practice in social work and probation, in Evidence-Based Practice: A Critical Appraisal. Edited by Trinder L, Reynolds S. Oxford, UK, Blackwell Scientific, 2000b, pp 138–162

Trinder L: Introduction: the context of evidence-based practice, in Evidence-Based Practice: A Critical Appraisal. Edited by Trinder L, Reynolds S. Oxford, UK, Blackwell Scientific, 2000c, pp 1–16

U.S. Department of Health and Human Services: Mental Health: A Report of the Surgeon General. Washington, DC, U.S. Department of Health and Human Services, 1999

Williams DDR, Garner J: The case against 'the evidence': a different perspective on evidence-based medicine. Br J Psychiatry 180:8–12, 2002

Young AS, Klap R, Sherbourne C, et al: The quality of care for depressive and anxiety disorders in the United States. Arch Gen Psychiatry 58:55–63, 2001

2

THE 5-STEP EVIDENCE-BASED MEDICINE MODEL

Although the philosophy of evidence-based medicine (EBM) can be rather abstract and sometimes even controversial, the basic strategy and methods of EBM are quite straightforward. EBM involves the application of a 5-step model (Table 2–1) to apply evidence from the medical literature to patient care problems (Gray 2002; Sackett et al. 2000). Details of this model are provided in Chapters 3–12 of this guide.

■ STEP 1: FORMULATE THE QUESTION

The EBM process begins with a clinical question, which may involve issues related to the diagnosis, treatment, prognosis, or etiology of a patient's illness. As described in Chapter 3, the question is formatted to include a patient problem or diagnosis; the treatment, diagnostic test, risk factor, or prognostic factor of interest, as well as any comparison; and the outcome of interest.

TABLE 2–1. **The 5-step evidence-based medicine process**

Step 1: Formulate the question
Step 2: Search for answers
Step 3: Appraise the evidence
Step 4: Apply the results
Step 5: Assess the outcome

■ STEP 2: SEARCH FOR ANSWERS

After formulating the question, the next step is to try to find an answer in the literature. This step involves an assessment of the type of evidence that is most appropriate for answering the question as well as the actual search for the evidence. Details of both processes can be found in Chapter 4.

■ STEP 3: APPRAISE THE EVIDENCE

After an article has been located, it is necessary to appraise its validity and importance before applying the results. The specific questions to ask regarding validity and importance depend on the type of study design and the nature of the question. In addition, you must decide whether the results can be applied to your particular patient and in your setting. The appraisal process is described in detail in Chapters 5–11.

■ STEP 4: APPLY THE RESULTS TO YOUR PATIENT

Assuming that the evidence you have found is valid, important, applicable to your patient, and feasible in your setting, the next step is to apply it to the care of your patient, which is where your clinical expertise is most important.

■ STEP 5: ASSESS THE OUTCOME

Step 5 includes an evaluation of your performance in searching the literature and in finding an answer to the clinical question posed, as well as an assessment of the patient's response to your treatment. Details of this step can be found in Chapter 12.

■ SOME SHORTCUTS

Studies in academic settings have found that the full 5-step model can be incorporated into routine practice (Ball 1998; Del Mar and Glasziou 2001; Sackett et al. 2000). In nonacademic settings, however, practitioners frequently voice concerns that are related to lack of time and information resources, as well as to an inadequate knowledge of the EBM process (Ely et al. 2002; Haines and Donald 1998; Lipman 2000; McColl et al. 1998; Straus and McAlister 2000; Trinder 2000; Young and Ward 2001).

There are, however, several shortcuts that can be taken to streamline the process and to make it more practical in everyday clinical practice. First, it is important to recognize that a clinician does not have to go through the 5-step process for every patient encounter (Sackett et al. 2000; Straus and McAlister 2000). After a question has been researched for one patient with a particular diagnosis, the answer can be applied to similar patients with the same diagnosis. In addition, because most patients of most psychiatrists fall into relatively few diagnostic categories, it soon becomes the exceptional patient who triggers the application of the full 5-step process.

One way to keep track of the results of a previous search and of the appraisal of an article is to summarize the paper in a structured format, which is referred to as a *critically appraised topic* (CAT) (Badenoch 2002; Badenoch and Heneghan 2002; Sackett et al. 2000). Examples of CATs can be found at the Duke University Medical Center Psychiatry and Behavioral Sciences Web site (http://psychiatry.mc.duke.edu/Residents/Quest.html). There is even software available that can store your summary in a uniform format (Badenoch n.d.). However, it is important to realize that the medical literature does change over time; therefore, you may need to repeat the search and appraisal process periodically, as new research becomes available. This is particularly important if new therapies or diagnostic procedures are being introduced for a diagnosis of interest.

As is discussed in more detail in Chapter 4, another way to

simplify the process is to use preappraised information resources, such as *Clinical Evidence* and *Evidence-Based Mental Health*. These resources allow practitioners to quickly search a database that is limited to high-quality preappraised evidence. Doing so makes the search process (step 2) much faster and eliminates the need to critically appraise the evidence (step 3). With access to on-line databases, such as *Clinical Evidence* and *Evidence-Based Mental Health*, information can be accessed quite quickly in the office, often in the same amount of time it would take to look something up in a conventional textbook (Gray 2002; Haynes 2001; Haynes et al. 2000; Tomlin 2000). For those without Internet access, print versions of *Clinical Evidence*, which are updated every 6 months, are available.

A third way to simplify the EBM process is through the use of a clinical informatics service provided either by a medical librarian or by a clinician skilled in EBM (Davidoff and Florance 2000; Greenhalgh et al. 2002). In this case, the clinician formulates a clinical question and submits it to the informatics service, which then returns an answer based on the best available evidence. This model has previously been implemented in academic medical centers, as well as in general practice settings, and is now being tried in inner-city public mental health clinic settings (G.E. Gray, unpublished data, June 2002).

Despite these shortcuts, there still will be questions that cannot be readily answered by the results of a previous search (stored as a CAT) or by the use of preappraised information resources. It is important therefore that psychiatrists and other clinicians be able to carry out the full 5-step EBM process when necessary (Evans 2001; Gray 2002; Guyatt et al. 2000; Haynes 2001; Straus et al. 2002).

■ REFERENCES

Badenoch D: Catmaker [Centre for Evidence-Based Medicine Web site]. n.d. Available at: http://www.cebm.net/catmaker.asp. Accessed June 27, 2003

Badenoch D: What is a CAT? [Centre for Evidence-Based Medicine website]. May 31, 2002. Available at: http://www.cebm.net/cat_ about.asp. Accessed June 27, 2003

Badenoch D, Heneghan C: Evidence-Based Medicine Toolkit. London, BMJ Books, 2002

Ball C: Evidence-based medicine on the wards: report from an evidence-based minion. Evidence-Based Medicine 3:101–103, 1998

Davidoff F, Florance V: The informationist: a new health profession? Ann Int Med 132:996–998, 2000

Del Mar CB, Glasziou PP: Ways of using evidence-based medicine in general practice. Med J Aust 174:347–350, 2001

Ely JW, Osheroff JA, Ebell MH, et al: Obstacles to answering doctors' questions about patient care with evidence: qualitative study. BMJ 324:710–713, 2002

Evans M: Creating knowledge management skills in primary care residents: a description of a new pathway to evidence-based practice in the community. Evidence-Based Medicine 6:133–34, 2001

Gray GE: Evidence-based medicine: an introduction for psychiatrists. J Psychiatr Pract 8:5–13, 2002

Greenhalgh T: How to Read a Paper: The Basics of Evidence Based Medicine, 2nd Edition. London, BMJ Books, 2001

Greenhalgh T, Hughes J, Humphrey C, et al: A comparative case study of two models of a clinical informaticist service. BMJ 324:524–529, 2002

Guyatt GH, Meade MO, Jaeschke RZ, et al: Practitioners of evidence based care. BMJ 320:954–955, 2000

Haines A, Donald A: Getting research findings into practice: making better use of research findings. BMJ 317:72–75, 1998

Haynes RB: Of studies, summaries, synopses and systems: the "4S" evolution of services for finding current best evidence. Evid Based Ment Health 4:37–39, 2001

Haynes RB, Glasziou P, Straus S: Advances in evidence-based information resources for clinical practice. ACP J Club 132:A11–A14, 2000

Lipman T: Evidence-based practice in general practice and primary care, in Evidence-Based Practice: A Critical Appraisal. Edited by Trinder L, Reynolds S. Oxford, Blackwell Scientific, 2000, pp 35–65

McColl A, Smith H, White P, et al: General practitioners' perception of the route to evidence based medicine: a questionnaire study. BMJ 316:361–365, 1998

Sackett DL, Strauss SE, Richardson WS, et al: Evidence-Based Medicine: How to Practice and Teach EBM, 2nd Edition. New York, Churchill Livingstone, 2000

Straus SE, McAlister FA: Evidence-based medicine: a commentary on common criticisms. CMAJ 163:837–841, 2000

Straus S, McAlister F, Cook D, et al: Expanded philosophy of evidence-based medicine: criticisms of evidence-based medicine, in Users' Guides to the Medical Literature: A Manual for Evidence-Based Clinical Care. Edited by Guyatt G, Rennie D. Chicago, IL, AMA Press, 2002, pp 211–222

Tomlin A: Answering mental health questions with reliable research evidence. Evid Based Ment Health 3:6–7, 2000

Trinder L: A critical appraisal of evidence-based practice, in Evidence-Based Practice: A Critical Appraisal. Edited by Trinder L, Reynolds S. Oxford, Blackwell Scientific, 2000, pp 212–241

Young JM, Ward JE: Evidence-based medicine in general practice: beliefs and barriers among Australian GPs. J Eval Clin Pract 7:201–210, 2001

3

ASKING ANSWERABLE
QUESTIONS

Every clinical encounter generates questions. Some of these require information that can be obtained only from the patient or from a collateral source, such as a friend or family member. Answers to such questions are unique to the particular patient and concern that patient's illness or situation. These types of questions form the basis of a psychiatric interview and are not the subject of this chapter.

■ BACKGROUND QUESTIONS VERSUS FOREGROUND QUESTIONS

This chapter focuses on questions about a patient's illness that are more general and hence answerable in the psychiatric literature. Such questions are often divided into two categories: background and foreground questions (McKibbon et al. 2002; Sackett et al. 2000).

Background questions concern relatively well-established facts. These are the sorts of questions that are best answered by reference books or textbooks. Examples of background questions are:

• *What are the DSM-IV-TR diagnostic criteria for panic disorder?*
• *What are the dosage forms for olanzapine?*
• *What is cognitive behavior therapy?*

Such questions typically have two parts: the journalistic "who, what, where, why, and how" and the name of a disorder or therapy.

Background questions are the types of questions that medical students and beginning residents most frequently ask.

Foreground questions, in contrast, concern the current best information on diagnosis, treatment, or prognosis of a disorder. Such questions are best answered by the research literature, not by textbooks, because they concern information that is still in a state of flux as new knowledge is accumulated. Foreground questions are the most frequent type of questions generated by senior residents or by practicing clinicians.

■ THE 4-PART QUESTION

Foreground questions are best framed as a 4-part question (Table 3–1). The question should include the patient(s) or problem of interest; the intervention of interest, including any comparison group; and the outcome of interest (Badenoch and Heneghan 2002; Dawes 1999; Geddes 1999; McKibbon et al. 2002; Sackett et al. 2000). Such questions are sometimes referred to as PICO questions (i.e., questions that use the mnemonic aid "**p**atient/problem, **i**ntervention, **c**omparison, and **o**utcome") (Gray 2002). A question formulated in this way provides the parameters needed to conduct an efficient literature search, because it makes the type of information required very clear.

TABLE 3–1. **The 4-part PICO question**

P: Patient or problem of interest

I: Intervention of interest
        Treatment
        Diagnostic test
        Risk factor
        Prognostic factor

C: Comparison
        Implicit or explicit

O: Outcome of interest
        Positive or negative

Patients or Problem

The first part of the question involves the patients or problem of interest. The degree of specificity has an influence on your ability to find an answer, as well as on the applicability of that answer to the particular patient of interest to you. Because you will be using the 4-part question as the starting point for your literature search, the patient or problem should be defined with a degree of specificity consistent with the way that study populations are defined. For example, if you are interested in the treatment of depression in preadolescents, specifying your population as "preadolescents with major depression" is preferable to "patients with major depression" because there are reasons to believe that the response to treatment might be different. However, if you become overly specific and specify "9-year-old Latino girls with a first episode of major depression and with a paternal—but not maternal—history of recurrent major depression," you may not be able to find evidence that is specific to such a narrowly defined population.

Intervention and Comparison

Intervention can be a treatment or a diagnostic test. Loosely defined, it can also refer to a risk factor or prognostic factor. In most cases, the intervention of interest will be compared with another intervention; in some cases, the comparison is explicit.

For questions related to treatment, the intervention can be either a specific medication or a psychosocial intervention. The comparison can be another active treatment, a placebo, or "usual care."

Diagnostic questions are usually questions related to the performance of a diagnostic test, screening instrument, or rating scale. The performance is usually compared with either a diagnostic "gold standard" or a commonly used instrument. Details of such comparisons are given in Chapter 8.

For questions related to etiology, the "intervention" is actually a risk factor. Here the comparison is often implicit (i.e., the absence of that risk factor).

Questions related to prognosis may be either 3- or 4-part questions. A 3-part question might ask the prognosis of patients with first-episode schizophrenia in general, whereas a 4-part question might ask whether a particular patient characteristic (prognostic factor) alters the prognosis. Here, as in questions related to etiology, the comparison can be implicit (i.e., the absence of the particular prognostic factor).

Outcome(s)

The fourth part of the question relates to the outcome or outcomes of interest. Such outcomes can be either positive (clinical improvement, remission, or survival) or negative (relapse, self-injury, or death). For questions involving diagnosis, the outcome is a measure of agreement between the two diagnostic methods.

Examples of 4-Part PICO Questions

Treatment

An example of a 4-part question related to treatment is

- *In adult patients with schizophrenia, does the addition of cognitive behavior therapy to usual care, compared with usual care alone, prevent relapse?*

In this example, the patients are "adult patients with schizophrenia," the intervention is the "addition of cognitive behavior therapy to usual care," the comparison is "usual care alone," and the outcome is "relapse."

Diagnosis

An example of a 4-part question related to diagnosis is

- *In a primary care clinic population, is the self-administration of a brief screening instrument as effective in identifying patients with major depression as is a structured brief clinical interview by a psychiatrist?*

In this example, the patients are "a primary care clinic population," the intervention (diagnostic test) is a self-administered brief screening instrument, the comparison (i.e., the "gold standard") is a structured brief clinical interview by a psychiatrist, and the outcome is a diagnosis of major depression.

Etiology/Harm

An example of a 4-part question related to etiology is

* *Among rescue workers at the site of the World Trade Center disaster, does the amount of time working at the disaster site influence the risk of developing posttraumatic stress disorder?*

In this example, the population of interest is "rescue workers at the site of the World Trade Center disaster," the intervention (risk factor) is "the amount of time working at the disaster site," the comparison is implicit (i.e., less time vs. more time), and the outcome is the onset of posttraumatic stress disorder.

A different type of question related to harm, this time with an explicit comparison group, is

* *In elderly patients (ages 65 years and older) with schizophrenia receiving maintenance therapy with an antipsychotic medication, are patients receiving olanzapine at less risk of developing tardive dyskinesia than patients receiving risperidone?*

In this example, the patients are "elderly patients (ages 65 years and older) with schizophrenia," the treatment of interest is olanzapine, the comparison treatment is risperidone, and the outcome of interest is the development of tardive dyskinesia.

Prognosis

An example of a 4-part question related to prognosis is

- *In patients ages 15–45 years, do female patients have better social and vocational functioning than male patients after experi-
  encing their first episode of schizophrenia?*

In this example, the patients are ages 15–45 years and have experienced their first episode of schizophrenia, the intervention (prognostic factor) is being female, the comparison group is male
patients, and the outcome is social and vocational functioning. Had
the question not explicitly asked about differences between male
and female patients, it would have been an equally acceptable 3-part
prognostic question.

■ REFERENCES

Badenoch D, Heneghan C: Evidence-Based Medicine Toolkit. London,
    BMJ Books, 2002

Dawes M: Formulating a question, in Evidence-Based Practice: A Primer
    for Health Professionals. Edited by Dawes M, Davies P, Gray A, et al.
    New York, Churchill Livingstone, 1999, pp 9–13

Geddes J: Asking structured and focused clinical questions: essential first
    step of evidence-based practice. Evid Based Ment Health 2:35–36, 1999

Gray GE: Evidence-based medicine: an introduction for psychiatrists. J Psy-
    chiatr Pract 8:5–13, 2002

McKibbon A, Hunt D, Richardson WS, et al: Finding the evidence, in Us-
    ers' Guides to the Medical Literature: A Manual for Evidence-Based
    Clinical Care. Edited by Guyatt G, Rennie D. Chicago, IL, AMA Press,
    2002, pp 13–47

Sackett DL, Strauss SE, Richardson WS, et al: Evidence-Based Medicine:
    How to Practice and Teach EBM, 2nd Edition. New York, Churchill Liv-
    ingstone, 2000

4

SEARCHING FOR ANSWERS

After formulating a 4-part PICO question (patient/problem, intervention, comparison, and outcome), the next step in the evidence-based medicine (EBM) process is to search for the best evidence to answer it. However, before beginning a search for an answer to a clinical question, it is important to understand the nature of the question and the type of evidence that would best answer it.

■ WHAT TYPE OF EVIDENCE IS BEST?

Although most clinicians would view a randomized controlled trial (RCT) as the ideal ("gold standard") study design, this is primarily true for questions involving treatment efficacy. In fact, a variety of other study designs may be preferred if the question is one regarding etiology, harm, prognosis, or diagnosis (Geddes 1999; Greenhalgh 2001; McKibbon et al. 2002). Table 4–1 lists the preferred study designs for a number of different categories of clinical questions. As can be seen, a cohort study is a more appropriate design for questions relating to etiology, whereas diagnostic tests are best assessed in a cross-sectional study.

There are also generally agreed-upon hierarchies of evidence that indicate that certain types of research results should be given more weight than other types (Badenoch and Heneghan 2002; Geddes 1999; Phillips et al. 2001). The specific hierarchy depends on the type of clinical question being asked. Table 4–2 presents the evidence hierarchy for studies of therapy or harm. Types of evidence higher in the hierarchy are more apt to give a valid and unbiased es-

TABLE 4–1. **Matching the study design to the question**

Type of question	Preferred study design
Diagnosis	Cross-sectional study
Treatment	Randomized controlled trial
Prognosis	Cohort study
Etiology or harm	Cohort or case-control study

Source. Adapted from Gray 2002.

TABLE 4–2. **Hierarchy of evidence for studies of therapy or harm**

Quality	Type of evidence
1a (best)	Systematic review of RCTs
1b	Individual RCT with narrow confidence interval
1c	"All-or-none" case series (see p. 53)
2a	Systematic review of cohort studies
2b	Individual cohort study
	RCT with <80% follow-up
2c	Outcomes research
	Ecological study
3a	Systematic review of case-control studies
3b	Individual case-control study
4	Case series
5 (worst)	Expert opinion

Note. RCT=randomized controlled trial.
Source. Adapted from Gray 2002; Phillips et al. 2001; Sackett et al. 2000.

timate of the effect of an intervention than are those lower in the hierarchy. When attempting to answer a clinical question, you should always rely on the evidence you have found that is highest in the hierarchy. It should be noted that expert opinion falls at the bottom of this hierarchy; therefore, expert opinion may be the basis for a clinical decision when no other evidence is available.

These hierarchies of evidence have been validated by comparing results obtained from studies that addressed the same question but used different designs. In studies of a variety of therapies, for example, it has repeatedly been shown that observational studies may give misleading results compared with RCTs (Lacchetti and Guyatt 2002). Whether the observational studies over- or underestimate the effectiveness of a particular treatment or preventive practice depends on the specific intervention being considered (Reeves et al. 2001). Expert opinion falls at the bottom, because such opinion does not necessarily reflect the best evidence found in the current research literature (Antman et al. 1992).

As an example of the use of an evidence hierarchy for questions related to treatment (Table 4–2), results from a systematic review of RCTs should be given more weight than the results of a single RCT, and results from an RCT should be given more weight than results from uncontrolled or nonexperimental studies. Thus, if your literature search produces a systematic review of RCTs, several individual RCTs, case reports, and an editorial, you should rely on the systematic review because it is highest in the evidence hierarchy.

■ THE "4S" APPROACH TO SEARCHING FOR ANSWERS

After the question has been categorized and the appropriate type of evidence required has been identified, the clinician can begin to search for an answer. Although many clinicians begin their search with *MEDLINE*, this is a relatively inefficient strategy because it typically identifies a large number of articles that must then be individually reviewed for validity. A more efficient approach is the hierarchical "4S" strategy of Haynes (2001a, 2001b), which involves *systems, synopses, syntheses,* and *studies* (Table 4–3). In this strategy, priority is given to sources of high-quality, preappraised information so that the clinician can omit the appraisal step (step 3) in the EBM process. In addition, this strategy favors brief summaries over lengthier reviews, assuming that a busy clinician wants an answer as quickly and effortlessly as possible. Although this strategy is appropriate for quickly answering clinical questions in a practice setting, it is not necessarily the most appropriate strategy for performing a comprehensive search of the clinical literature.

■ SYSTEMS

The starting point for the search should be what Haynes (2001a, 2001b) has termed a *system*, an information source that covers a variety of diagnoses, provides a summary of the results of high-quality systematic reviews, and is frequently updated. Such a system would provide the user with a concise summary of the evidence, linked to the original studies.

There are currently several information sources that fit Haynes's definition of systems: *Clinical Evidence*, the National electronic Library for Mental Health (NeLMH), and several collections of clinical practice guidelines. Each source has advantages and disadvantages, which are described below.

Clinical Evidence

Clinical Evidence is published semiannually by the BMJ Publishing Group (Barton 2001a, 2001b). It consists of chapters on 145 topics, including several psychiatric disorders (Alzheimer's disease, anorexia nervosa, attention deficit hyperactivity disorder, bulimia nervosa, depression in children and adults, generalized anxiety disorder, obsessive-compulsive disorder, panic disorder, posttraumatic stress disorder, and schizophrenia). Each chapter includes summaries on several different therapies. The chapter on depressive disorders, for example, begins with a table outlining which interventions are and are not effective, followed by summaries of three classes of antidepressants, electroconvulsive therapy, four psychotherapies, combined (antidepressant plus psychotherapy) treatment, and several other therapies (Geddes and Butler 2002). For each type of therapy, there is a summary of benefits and side effects, followed by a more detailed review of the literature, with references to systematic reviews and to RCTs. Thus, the reader

TABLE 4-3. **The 4S approach to searching for answers**

Type of information resource	Examples	Web site
Systems (comprehensive sources)	*Clinical Evidence*	http://www.clinicalevidence.com
	National electronic Library for Mental Health	http://www.nelmh.org
	APA practice guidelines	http://www.psych.org/clin_res/prac_guide.cfm
Synopses (structured abstracts)	*Evidence-Based Mental Health*	http://ebmh.bmjjournals.com
	ACP Journal Club	http://www.acpjc.org/
Syntheses (systematic reviews)	*Cochrane Database of Systematic Reviews*	http://www.update-software.com/abstracts/mainindex.htm
	Database of Abstracts of Effectiveness (DARE)	http://nhscrd.york.ac.uk/darehp.htm
Studies (original articles)	*MEDLINE (PubMed)*	http://www.ncbi.nlm.nih.gov:80/entrez/query/static/clinical.html

Source. Adapted from Gray 2002; Haynes 2001a, 2001b.

progresses from a brief overview to progressively more detailed information and references. *Clinical Evidence* is a work in progress; additional disorders and treatments are added with each issue (Barton 2001a, 2001b).

In addition to the original print version of *Clinical Evidence*, there is also a shorter specialty version that contains only the mental health sections (Clinical Evidence 2002b). This version is more portable and less expensive than the original and is also updated semiannually.

Clinical Evidence is also available online (by subscription) at http://www.clinicalevidence.com or through the Ovid database collection at http://www.ovid.com, to which many medical libraries have subscriptions (Etchells 2000; Polmear 2000). In addition, *Clinical Evidence* may be downloaded to a personal digital assistant by using the CogniQ platform (Clinical Evidence 2002).

Because of its ease of use, frequent updates, multiple platforms, and clear linkage to the best evidence, *Clinical Evidence* should generally be the starting point for a search; however, there are several alternative systems.

National electronic Library for Mental Health

The NeLMH (http://www.nelmh.org), a "virtual branch library" within the National electronic Library for Health (NeLH) (http://www.nelh.nhs.uk), is part of the National Health Service (NHS) Information for Health Strategy (NHS Information Authority 2001). The NeLH is an ambitious effort to provide health professionals with access to a variety of evidence-based resources (NeLH 2002). There are several such virtual branch libraries with specialty-specific content, including the NeLMH.

The NeLMH was created by the Centre for Evidence-Based Mental Health (2001a, 2002) and is described in detail by Dearness and Tomlin (2001). The site currently provides information about only three topics (depression, schizophrenia, and suicide), although there are plans to expand the content. For a given topic, there is information about diagnosis (including both DSM-IV-TR [American

Psychiatric Association 2000] and ICD-10 criteria) and a variety of treatment options. For a given treatment option, there is a summary of evidence regarding effectiveness and side effects, linked to systematic reviews and RCTs. There are also links to relevant clinical guidelines.

Although the NeLMH is incomplete in terms of diagnoses, the information on the site is excellent. For questions related to schizophrenia, depression, or suicide, it can be a good starting point for your information search. As the NeLMH grows, it may well prove to be the model system.

Clinical Practice Guidelines

A third system is a collection of high-quality clinical practice guidelines (Guyatt et al. 2002). This section describes some collections of guidelines that may be useful starting points for questions regarding the treatment of mental disorders. General information about clinical practice guidelines can be found in Chapter 7.

American Psychiatric Association Practice Guidelines

Most American psychiatrists are familiar with the practice guidelines developed by the American Psychiatric Association (APA). These guidelines currently cover the major psychiatric disorders and are available both in print form (APA 2002b) and online (http://www.psych.org/clin_res/prac_guide.cfm).

Other Clinical Practice Guidelines

A variety of other organizations have also produced high-quality clinical practice guidelines that may be useful starting points in answering clinical questions (Table 4–4). The most useful starting point in searching for these guidelines is the National Guideline Clearinghouse (http://www.guideline.gov). This database of clinical practice guidelines is operated by the Agency for Healthcare Research and Quality (AHRQ), in association with the American Medical Association and the American Association of Health

TABLE 4–4. Sources of high-quality clinical practice guidelines

Organization	Web site
American Psychiatric Association	http://www.psych.org/clin_res/prac_guide.cfm
National Guideline Clearinghouse	http://www.guideline.gov
Canadian Medical Association	http://mdm.ca/cpgsnew/cpgs/index.asp
New Zealand Guidelines Group	http://www.nzgg.org.nz/library.cfm
Prodigy (U.K. National Health Service)	http://www.prodigy.nhs.uk/ClinicalGuidance/ReleasedGuidance/GuidanceList.asp
Scottish Intercollegiate Guidelines Network	http://www.sign.ac.uk/guidelines/index.html

Plans. All guidelines must meet explicit quality criteria for inclusion (AHRQ 2000). Searching the database yields a structured abstract that is linked to the actual guideline. The database also allows several guidelines to be compared side by side.

■ SYNOPSES

If the system you have searched (NeLMH, *Clinical Evidence*, or a collection of practice guidelines) does not produce a result, the next step is to search for what Haynes (2001a, 2001b) has termed *synopses*, structured abstracts of high-quality systematic reviews or original articles. The advantages of these resources are that they have already been appraised for quality and are summarized; therefore, busy clinicians can quickly get to the bottom line without reading a lengthy article. Furthermore, these synopses can be accessed through online databases that can be searched quickly. Because these databases contain summaries of only those articles that meet certain quality criteria, they are much smaller than *MEDLINE* and yield fewer references.

Evidence-Based Mental Health

For psychiatry, the best source of synopses is *Evidence-Based Mental Health*, published quarterly by the BMJ Publishing Group. The online version (http://.ebmh.bmjjournals.com) is particularly useful in searching for answers to clinical questions related to common psychiatric disorders.

The staff at *Evidence-Based Mental Health* reviews the major medical and psychiatric journals to identify both original research articles and literature reviews that meet explicit quality criteria. They then prepare structured abstracts, sometimes reanalyzing the data to present it in a uniform format. An outside reviewer supplies a commentary. Finally, a declarative title summarizes the article's "clinical bottom line."

ACP Journal Club

ACP Journal Club, a publication that is similar to *Evidence-Based Mental Health*, is published bimonthly by the American College of Physicians–American Society of Internal Medicine and is available online (http://www.acpjc.org/). Although the intended audience is internists, *ACP Journal Club* does include summaries of articles of psychiatric interest that are related primarily to disorders seen in primary care settings (e.g., depression, anxiety disorders, dementia, delirium, and substance abuse). If you do not have access to *Evidence-Based Mental Health,* then searching the (free) *ACP Journal Club* database may prove useful.

Best Evidence

Best Evidence is available through many medical libraries as one of the Ovid databases (http://www.ovid.com). It consists of the combined contents of *ACP Journal Club* and a sister British publication, *Evidence-Based Medicine* (Davidoff et al. 1995; McKibbon et al. 2002). As with the online *ACP Journal Club*, the psychiatric content is not as extensive as *Evidence-Based Mental Health*, but it may still have an answer to your question.

■ SYNTHESES

If a relevant synopsis cannot be found, the next step is to search for what Haynes (2001a, 2001b) has termed a *synthesis*, a high-quality systematic review. A detailed discussion of systematic reviews and how they are appraised for quality is given in Chapter 6. The following discussion concentrates on the methods used for locating systematic reviews.

Cochrane Database of Systematic Reviews

The single best source of systematic reviews is the *Cochrane Database of Systematic Reviews* (Glanville and Lefebvre 2000; McKibbon et al. 2002). This database contains high-quality systematic reviews specially prepared by the Cochrane Collaborative, a multi-site international workgroup (Antes and Oxman 2001; Cochrane Collaboration 1997). The full-text version of the reviews is available through medical libraries as part of their Ovid database subscription (http://www.ovid.com). Abstracts of the reviews are available online (without charge) from the Update Software Web site (http://www.update-software.com/ abstracts/mainindex.htm), and the full-text version may be ordered at this Web site for a fee.

Database of Abstracts of Reviews of Effectiveness

The *Database of Abstracts of Reviews of Effectiveness* (*DARE*) consists of structured abstracts of systematic reviews that meet certain quality criteria (NHS Centre for Reviews and Dissemination [NHS CRD] 2000). *DARE* is maintained by the NHS CRD at the University of York and can be accessed through their Web site (http://nhscrd.york.ac.uk/darehp.htm). *DARE* is also available through medical libraries as part of Ovid's *Evidence-Based Medicine Reviews*, a database that combines *Best Evidence*, the *Cochrane Database of Systematic Reviews*, and *DARE* (Etchells 2000; Ovid 2002b). Because *DARE* provides only abstracts of reviews, the actual review must be obtained separately if further detail is required.

Health Technology Assessment Database

The *Health Technology Assessment* (*HTA*) database (http://nhscrd.york.ac.uk/htahp.htm) is also maintained by the NHS CRD at the University of York, in collaboration with the International Network of Agencies for Health Technology Assessment (INAHTA) (NHS CRD 2002). It contains abstracts of critical reviews of health technologies, including treatments for psychiatric conditions. Most of the abstracts are linked to the Web site of the agency that produces the report, from which the full text of the document can be obtained. The *HTA* and *DARE* databases may be searched simultaneously from the NHS CRD Web site (http://144.32.228.3/scripts/WEBC.EXE/NHSCRD/start).

Other Sources of Systematic Reviews

Several other organizations produce high-quality systematic reviews. Some of the major sources that provide online access to their reviews are listed in Table 4–5.

Systematic reviews published in journals may also be identified through *MEDLINE* and similar databases. This can be accomplished most efficiently with the assistance of "filters" that attempt to limit the search results to systematic reviews or meta-analyses (Glanville and Lefebvre 2000; McKibbon et al. 1999; NHS CRD 2002; Shojania and Berg 2001). This process is described in more detail in the next section.

■ STUDIES

You would search *MEDLINE* or similar databases only if you had been unsuccessful in finding an answer to your clinical question using the resources in the first three *S*'s of the 4S approach. This is because such a search is apt to yield multiple studies that you would then have to appraise. In contrast, the resources described in the first three categories are sources of high-quality evidence that have generally already been preappraised for validity, thus sparing you the need to go through the critical-appraisal step before using the evidence.

There are multiple databases that can be useful in locating answers to mental health–related questions. However, much of the focus of this section is placed on *MEDLINE*, partly because psychiatrists are generally most familiar with this resource and can access it most readily. In addition, there is empirical evidence that *MEDLINE* is more apt to be useful in identifying results of psychotherapy studies than are *Excerpta Medica* (*EMBASE*) or *PsycINFO* (Watson and Richardson 1999a, 1999b).

MEDLINE

MEDLINE is a database maintained by the U.S. National Library of Medicine (NLM). It includes over 11 million citations, both clinical

TABLE 4-5. Sources of high-quality systematic reviews

Organization or database	Web site
Cochrane Database of Systematic Reviews	http://www.update-software.com/abstracts/mainindex.htm
Database of Abstracts of Reviews of Effectiveness	http://nhscrd.york.ac.uk/darehp.htm
Health Technology Assessment Database	http://nhscrd.york.ac.uk/htahp.htm
Agency for Healthcare Research and Quality	http://www.ahcpr.gov/clinic/epc/
Canadian Coordination Office for Health Technology Assessment	http://www.ccohta.ca/entry_e.html
Centre for Clinical Effectiveness at Monash University (Australia)	http://www.med.monash.edu.au/healthservices/cce/evidence/
National Health Service Centre for Reviews and Dissemination (United Kingdom)	http://www.york.ac.uk/inst/crd/ehcb.htm

and preclinical (McKibbon et al. 2002). *MEDLINE* may be accessed through a variety of different services. Libraries usually obtain the *MEDLINE* database through a commercial vendor, such as Ovid or SilverPlatter. *MEDLINE* access is available free of charge, using the National Library of Medicine's *PubMed* Web site (http://www.ncbi.nlm.nih.gov/entrez/query.fcgi).

PubMed

For most psychiatrists, the simplest starting point for a *MEDLINE* search (using *PubMed*) is the Clinical Queries interface (http://www.ncbi.nlm.nih.gov/entrez/query/static/clinical.html) (Gray 2002; Zaroukian 2001). The Clinical Queries interface allows the user to specify the type of question (therapy, diagnosis, etiology, or prognosis) and whether the search will be sensitive or specific. *PubMed* then applies search filters to limit the search to particular types of articles. This filtering is achieved by addition of specific terms to the search, in addition to the terms that the user entered. Table 4–6 lists the search terms used in the *PubMed* filters, which were derived from the work of Haynes et al. (1994). Choosing *therapy* and *specificity*, for example, has *PubMed* search for articles with *double blind* or *placebo* in the title to limit the results to double-blind or placebo-controlled studies. Choosing *therapy* and *sensitivity* provides results that include RCTs, trials of drug therapy, therapeutic use of a drug, or studies that have *random* in the title. This will yield more articles; however, many of the articles will not actually include RCTs. The Clinical Queries interface also allows the user to search for systematic reviews using similar filters (Shojania and Berg 2001).

Ovid MEDLINE

Ovid is the supplier of *MEDLINE* to most medical libraries in the United States. The Ovid search interface allows the user to limit the search to specific types of articles or study designs (e.g., RCT, clinical trial, or Phase III clinical trial), as well as to search by text word

TABLE 4–6. *PubMed* Clinical Queries search filters

Type of question	Search filter for specificity	Search filter for sensitivity
Therapy	(double [WORD] AND blind* [WORD]) OR placebo [WORD]	"randomized controlled trial" [PTYP] OR "drug therapy: [SH] OR "therapeutic use" [SH:NOEXP] or "random*" [WORD]
Diagnosis	"sensitivity and specificity" [MeSH] OR ("predictive" [WORD] AND "value*" [WORD])	"sensitivity and specificity" [WORD] OR "sensitivity" [WORD] OR "diagnosis" [SH] or "diagnostic use" [SH] OR "specificity" [WORD]
Etiology	"case-control studies" [MH:NOEXP] OR "cohort studies" [MH:NOEXP]	"cohort studies" [MeSH] or "risk" [MeSH] OR ("odds" [WORD] AND "ratio*" [WORD]) OR ("relative" [WORD] AND "risk" [WORD]) OR "case-control*" [WORD] OR "case-control studies" [MeSH]
Prognosis	"prognosis" [MH:NOEXP] OR "survival analysis" [MH:NOEXP]	"incidence" [MeSH] OR "mortality" [MeSH] or "follow-up studies" [MeSH] or "mortality" [SH] OR "prognosis*" [WORD] OR "predict*" [WORD] OR "course" [WORD]

or medical subject heading (MeSH) term. Greenhalgh (1997, 2001) has authored excellent guides to efficiently searching the Ovid version of *MEDLINE*. In addition, McKibbon et al. (1999) have provided a thorough description of ways to use publication type, text words, and MeSHs to identify specific types of studies in the *MEDLINE* database. There are also several filters that can be used with *Ovid*, similar to the built-in filters in *PubMed* (Critical Appraisal Skills Programme 2002; London Library and Information Development Unit 2001a; University of Rochester Medical Center 2002b).

WinSPIRS MEDLINE

The other common supplier of the *MEDLINE* database to medical libraries is SilverPlatter, with its WinSPIRS version. Once again, there are filters available for this version of *MEDLINE* (London Library and Information Development Unit 2001b).

Other Databases

Although *MEDLINE* is usually the best starting point for a search, there are a variety of other specialized databases that may be useful in searching for particular types of evidence (Greenhalgh 2001; Snowball 1999). McKibbon et al. (1999) have provided useful guidance on searching for specific types of articles in these databases.

EMBASE, the Excerpta Medica Database

EMBASE is an international medical and pharmaceutical database that covers 3,600 publications from 70 countries (Greenhalgh 2001; Ovid 2002a; Snowball 1999). It is much like a European version of *MEDLINE* and it covers some European and non–English language journals that are not included in *MEDLINE*. Filters for *EMBASE* are available (Critical Appraisal Skills Programme 2002).

Cumulative Index to Nursing and Allied Health Literature

The *Cumulative Index to Nursing and Allied Health Literature* (*CINAHL*) covers 1,000 English-language nursing and allied health journals (Greenhalgh 2001; Ovid 2002a; Snowball 1999). Filters may be used to focus searches (Critical Skills Appraisal Programme 2002; University of Rochester Medical Center 2002a).

ClinPSYC and PsycINFO

ClinPSYC and *PsycINFO* are databases produced by the American Psychological Association (Greenhalgh 2001; Ovid 2002a; Snowball 1999). *PsycINFO* covers 1,800 journals in more than 25 languages. *ClinPSYC* is a clinically oriented subset of the *PsycINFO* database. Filters for *PsycINFO* are available (Critical Appraisal Skills Programme 2003).

■ ALTERNATIVES TO THE 4S APPROACH

The 4S approach by Haynes (2001a, 2001b) is a stepwise search strategy, beginning with systems and progressing until an answer to the clinical question is found. An alternative strategy is to simultaneously search several databases that include two or more levels in the hierarchy. Two search engines that perform this function are the *TRIP Database* and *SUMSearch*.

TRIP Database

The *TRIP Database* (http://www.tripdatabase.com) was created in 1997 and is currently the search engine for the NeLH. Updated monthly, it is an attempt to link all of the high-quality evidence-based resources available on the Internet. A search using the *TRIP Database* will search the *Cochrane Library*, *DARE*, other collections of systematic reviews and guidelines, and even some online journals. It also has links to the *PubMed* Clinical Queries search interface.

SUMSearch

SUMSearch (http://sumsearch.uthscsa.edu/searchform45.htm) was developed at the University of Texas Health Sciences Center at San

Antonio. It simultaneously searches *MEDLINE*, *DARE*, the *National Guidelines Clearinghouse* database, the *Merck Manual*, and *PubMed* (Badgett 2000; Booth and O'Rourke 2000). Unlike the *TRIP Database*, which offers the option of repeating the search in *PubMed*, *SUMSearch* automatically searches *PubMed*, as well as the other databases. As a result, searches with *SUMSearch* often take 1–2 minutes longer than other searches.

■ EXAMPLES OF SEARCHING FOR EVIDENCE USING VARIOUS APPROACHES

To demonstrate the 4S approach to searching for evidence, as well as the use of the *TRIP Database* and *SUMSearch*, two examples of clinical questions and their resulting search results are given below.

Example 1: Cognitive-Behavioral Therapy in Schizophrenia

* *In patients with schizophrenia, does the addition of cognitive-behavioral therapy (CBT) to usual treatment, compared with usual treatment alone, prevent relapse?*

4S Approach: The search required about 15 seconds to yield an answer. The starting point for this search was a system, *Clinical Evidence*. The table on the first page of the chapter on schizophrenia indicated that CBT was likely to be beneficial in preventing relapse. In the same chapter, the section on CBT stated that "limited evidence from RCTs suggests that cognitive behavioral therapy may reduce relapse rates" and referred to a *Cochrane* review (McIntosh and Lawrie 2001). Because *Clinical Evidence* provided an answer, it was not necessary to search any further. However, for the purpose of seeing what the other recommended systems would yield, the NeLMH (NeLMH 2002) and APA (APA 2002b) practice guidelines were searched. The NeLMH provided similar information to that in *Clinical Evidence* (Centre for Evidence-Based

Mental Health 2001b), whereas the APA guideline (APA 2002a) indicated that there were "encouraging clinical results" regarding CBT and referenced a book and several articles, but not the *Cochrane* review.

TRIP Database

The *TRIP Database* was searched using the terms "cognitive AND therapy AND schizophrenia." Two references were obtained: a *Cochrane* review and an RCT of CBT in schizophrenia published in the *Archives of General Psychiatry* (Sensky et al. 2000). In this example, the *TRIP Database* was equal to *Clinical Evidence* and the NeLMH in speed and ease of use. It yielded a result faster than looking through the APA guideline compendium (APA 2002b), where the results were indexed under "cognitive remediation and therapy" rather than under CBT.

SUMSearch

SUMSearch was searched using the terms "cognitive therapy AND schizophrenia." The search, which took about 90 seconds, retrieved 4 citations in the *Merck Manual*, 5 *Cochrane* or AHRQ systematic reviews, 10 practice guidelines, 20 possible systematic reviews from *PubMed*, and 40 original research articles from *PubMed*. Most of the citations were not relevant; however, the search identified 2 relevant practice guidelines (including the APA guideline [APA 2002a]), the *Cochrane* review, and 3 other review articles (which may or may not have been systematic reviews). In this example, both the 4S approach and the *TRIP Database* yielded an answer faster than *SUMSearch* (i.e., both required less search time and less weeding-out of irrelevant search results).

Example 2: Kava in Generalized Anxiety Disorder

- *In patients with generalized anxiety disorder, is kava extract more effective than a placebo in relieving symptoms of anxiety?*

4S Approach: The search started with a system (*Clinical Evidence*), but the section on generalized anxiety disorder did not mention kava as a treatment. Using the terms "kava AND anxiety," an online search of *Evidence-Based Mental Health* failed to yield any articles. Using the same terms, a search of the *DARE* database yielded 5 articles, including a *Cochrane* review and 1 other systematic review of the efficacy of kava in anxiety disorders (Pittler and Ernst 2000, 2002). Even though the system and synopses failed to yield an answer, the entire search still took only slightly more than 1 minute.

TRIP Database

The *TRIP Database* was searched using the terms "kava AND anxiety." Three references were obtained: the same two systematic review identified in *DARE* (Pittler and Ernst 2000, 2002) and an article in *BMJ* on hepatitis associated with kava. Because the *TRIP Database* searched multiple databases, it yielded a result in about 15 seconds, which was clearly faster than the 4S approach.

SUMSearch

SUMSearch was searched using the terms "kava AND anxiety." This time the search took slightly less than 1 minute, and 26 references were obtained, including 1 *Cochrane* review and 1 editorial, 8 possible reviews, and 16 original articles from *PubMed*. The same two systematic reviews identified in *DARE* were among these results (Pittler and Ernst 2000, 2002). Compared with the *TRIP Database* search, the search with *SUMSearch* took slightly longer, and more time to sift through the results was also required. Compared with the 4S approach, search results were obtained faster, but again, it was necessary to sort through the results; therefore, on balance, the time to reach an answer was actually longer.

■ COMPARISON AND RECOMMENDATIONS

After performing a number of similar searches using all three methods, I found that each of the approaches has certain advantages and disadvantages. Overall, I found *SUMSearch* to be less useful than either the *TRIP Database* or the 4S approach, because the search itself takes longer than the *TRIP Database* and is less focused than either of the latter approaches. If an answer can be obtained in *Clinical Evidence*, the 4S approach tends to be the fastest; if not, the *TRIP Database* is faster.

Based on these admittedly unsystematic and undoubtedly biased observations, I would recommend a modified 4S approach that depends on the availability of information resources (Table 4–7). This is a hierarchical approach in which it is not necessary to go through all four levels. Instead, the search can be stopped as soon as a suitable answer is obtained.

I would suggest beginning the search with *Clinical Evidence*, because many questions can be answered easily and quickly with this resource. Furthermore, it has the advantage of being available online and in print, and it can be downloaded to your personal digital assistant.

If online access to *Evidence-Based Mental Health* is available, I recommend searching this database next. It includes synopses of original research that have not yet been incorporated into a systematic review, and the information is presented in a format that will provide an answer quickly.

The third step in my search is either the Ovid *Evidence-Based Medicine Reviews* or the *TRIP Database*. Both include the *Cochrane Database of Systematic Reviews* and *DARE*. The Ovid database includes *ACP Journal Club*, allows access to the full text of the reviews, and is linked to the full text of several journals. The *TRIP Database* includes other collections of systematic reviews and guidelines and is linked to a different set of full-text online journals, but it provides only the abstracts of the reviews. The choice between the two will depend on personal preferences and is limited by the availability of Ovid within your setting.

The final step in my search would be *MEDLINE*. I personally prefer the *PubMed* version with its Clinical Queries interface, although the linkage with full-text articles in the Ovid journal collection may be a compelling reason to use the Ovid version instead.

TABLE 4–7. Suggested search strategy

Step	Resource	Web site
1	*Clinical Evidence*	http://www.clinicalevidence.com
2	*Evidence-Based Mental Health*	http://ebmh.bmjjournals.com
3	*TRIP Database*	http://www.tripdatabase.com
	OR	
	Ovid *Evidence-Based Medicine Reviews*	(available through medical libraries)
4	*PubMed* Clinical Queries	http://www.ncbi.nlm.nih.gov/entrez/query/static/clinical.html
	OR	
	Ovid *MEDLINE*	(available through medical libraries)

■ WHAT IF YOU CANNOT FIND AN ANSWER?

There are three general reasons for not finding an answer to a clinical question. The first reason has to do with the mechanics of the search process. Changing the search terms, searching by MeSH heading as well as text words, and other techniques described in more detail elsewhere (Greenhalgh 1997, 2001; McKibbon et al. 1999, 2002) may be of value if this is the case.

The second reason has to do with the nature of the question itself. Perhaps the patient population specified in the question is overly specific (see Chapter 3). Broadening the patient population in the question may result in the search yielding a possible answer. The problem then becomes one of deciding whether that answer can be generalized to your particular patient. This is a topic discussed in more detail in subsequent chapters.

The third reason for not finding an answer is that the evidence either does not exist or that the only evidence is relatively unreliable. The search strategies outlined above tend to find evidence that is high in the evidence hierarchy (Table 4–2). If such high-quality evidence does not exist, it is necessary to search for evidence lower in the hierarchy. This can be done through *PubMed,* by changing the search filters in the Clinical Queries interface from "specificity" to "sensitivity" or by doing a *MEDLINE* search without filters. Such strategies may result in lower-quality evidence, such as case series or case reports. In some cases, this may represent the best available evidence. Obtaining consultation is another option. Although expert opinion is at the bottom of the evidence hierarchy, it is still better than nothing. Finally, evidence-based medicine retains a place for clinical judgment (Haynes et al. 2002a, 2002b). In the absence of evidence from the literature, clinical judgment becomes even more important.

■ REFERENCES

Agency for Healthcare Research and Quality: The National Guideline Clearinghouse fact sheet [Agency for Healthcare Research and Quality Web site]. July 2000. Available at: http://www.ahcpr.gov/clinic/ngc-fact.htm. Accessed June 18, 2002

American Psychiatric Association: Diagnostic and Statistical Manual of Mental Disorders, 4th Edition, Text Revision. Washington, DC, American Psychiatric Association, 2000

American Psychiatric Association: Practice guideline for the treatment of patients with schizophrenia, in Practice Guidelines for the Treatment of Psychiatric Disorders: Compendium 2002. Washington, DC, American Psychiatric Association, 2002a, pp 349–461

American Psychiatric Association: Practice Guidelines for the Treatment of Psychiatric Disorders: Compendium 2002. Washington, DC, American Psychiatric Association, 2002b

Antes G, Oxman AD: The Cochrane Collaboration in the 20th century, in Systematic Reviews in Health Care: Meta-Analysis in Context. Edited by Egger M, Smith GD, Altman DG. London, BMJ Books, 2001, pp 447–458

Antman EM, Lau J, Kupelnick B, et al: A comparison of results of meta-analyses of randomized control trials and recommendations of clinical experts: treatments for myocardial infarction. JAMA 268:240–248, 1992

Badenoch D, Heneghan C: Evidence-Based Medicine Toolkit. London, BMJ Books, 2002

Badgett B: SUMSearch-details [SUMSearch Web site]. July 19, 2000. Available at: http://sumsearch.uthscsa.edu/details.htm. Accessed June 20, 2002

Barton S: Using clinical evidence. BMJ 322:503–504, 2001a

Barton S: Welcome to issue 6. Clinical Evidence 6:ix–xii, 2001b

Booth A, O'Rourke A: SUMSearch and PubMed: 2 Internet-based evidence-based medicine tools. ACP J Club 132:A16, 2000

Centre for Evidence-Based Mental Health: NeLMH background information [National electronic Library for Mental Health Web site]. July 14, 2001a. Available at: http://cebmh.warne.ox.ac.uk/cebmh/elmh/nelmh/background.html. Accessed June 18, 2002

Centre for Evidence-Based Mental Health: Schizophrenia: evidence-based treatment summaries: talking treatments: cognitive behavioural therapy: detailed [National electronic Library for Mental Health Web site]. September 3, 2001b. Available at: http://cebmh.warne.ox.ac.uk/cebmh/elmh/nelmh/schizophrenia/treatment/talking/cogbehaviour2.html. Accessed June 20, 2002

Centre for Evidence-Based Mental Health: National electronic Library for Mental Health [National electronic Library for Mental Health Web site]. March 19, 2002. Available at: http://cebmh.warne.ox.ac.uk/cebmh/elmh/nelmh/index.html. Accessed June 18, 2002

Clinical Evidence: Mental Health. London, BMJ Publishing Group, 2002

Clinical Evidence: Handheld ce [*Clinical Evidence* Web site]. 2003. Available at: http://www.clinicalevidence.com/lpBinCE/lpext.dll?f=templates&fn=main-h.htm&2.0. Accessed June 18, 2002

Cochrane Collaboration: The Cochrane Collaboration leaflet [Cochrane Collaboration Web site]. Available at: http://www.cochrane.org/cochrane/leaflet.htm. May 15, 2003. Accessed June 27, 2003

Critical Appraisal Skills Programme: Filters [Critical Appraisal Skills Programme Web site]. 2002. Available at: http://www.phru.org.uk/~casp/filters.htm#findingfilters. Accessed June 27, 2003

Davidoff F, Haynes B, Sackett D, et al: Evidence based medicine. BMJ 310:1085–1086, 1995

Dearness KL, Tomlin A: Development of the National electronic Library for Mental Health: providing evidence-based information for all. Health Info Libr J 18:167–174, 2001

Etchells E: Ovid. ACP J Club 132:A15, 2000

Geddes J: Asking structured and focused clinical questions: essential first step of evidence-based practice. Evid Ment Health 2:35–36, 1999

Geddes J, Butler R: Depressive disorders. Clinical Evidence 7:867–882, 2002

Glanville J, Lefebvre C: Identifying systematic reviews: key resources. Evid Based Ment Health 3:68–69, 2000

Gray GE: Evidence-based medicine: an introduction for psychiatrists. J Psychiatr Pract 8:5–13, 2002

Greenhalgh T: How to read a paper: the *Medline* database. BMJ 315:180–183, 1997

Greenhalgh T: How to Read a Paper: The Basics of Evidence Based Medicine, 2nd Edition. London, BMJ Books, 2001

Guyatt G, Haynes B, Jaeschke R, et al: Introduction: the philosophy of evidence-based medicine, in Users' Guides to the Medical Literature: A Manual for Evidence-Based Clinical Practice. Edited by Guyatt G, Rennie D. Chicago, IL, AMA Press, 2002, pp 3–12

Haynes RB: Of studies, summaries, synopses, and systems: the "4S" evolution of services for finding current best evidence. Evid Based Ment Health 4:37–39, 2001a

Haynes RB: Of studies, syntheses, synopses, and systems: the "4S" evolution of services for finding current best evidence. ACP J Club 134:A11–A13, 2001b

Haynes RB, Wilczynski N, McKibbon KA, et al: Developing optimal search strategies for detecting clinically sound studies in *MEDLINE*. J Am Med Inform Assoc 1:447–458, 1994

Haynes RB, Devereaux PJ, Guyatt GH: Clinical expertise in the era of evidence-based medicine and patient choice. ACP J Club 136:A11–A14, 2002a

Haynes RB, Devereaux PJ, Guyatt GH: Physicians' and patients' choices in evidence based practice. BMJ 324:1350, 2002b

Lacchetti C, Guyatt G: Therapy and validity: surprising results of randomized controlled trials, in Users' Guides to the Medical Literature: A Manual for Evidence-Based Clinical Care. Edited by Guyatt G, Rennie D. Chicago, IL, AMA Press, 2002, pp 13–47

London Library and Information Development Unit: Some methodological filters—Ovid [LondonLInKS Web site]. April 10, 2001a. Available at: http://www.londonlinks.ac.uk/evidence_strategies/ovid_filters.htm. Accessed June 19, 2002

London Library and Information Development Unit: Some methodological filters—WinSPIRS [LondonLInKS Web site]. April 10, 2001b. Available at: http://www.londonlinks.ac.uk/evidence_strategies/win_filters.htm. Accessed June 19, 2002

McIntosh A, Lawrie S: Schizophrenia. Clinical Evidence 6:776–797, 2001

McKibbon A, Eady A, Marks S: PDQ Evidence-Based Principles and Practice. Hamilton, ON, Canada, BC Decker, 1999

McKibbon A, Hunt D, Richardson WS, et al: Finding the evidence, in Users' Guides to the Medical Literature: A Manual for Evidence-Based Clinical Care. Edited by Guyatt G, Rennie D. Chicago, IL, AMA Press, 2002, pp 247–265

National electronic Library for Health: The knowledge and know-how platform [National electronic Library for Health Web site]. July 2002. Available at: http://www.nhsia.nhs.uk/nelh/pages/arch_knowledgeplat.asp. Accessed October 16, 2002

National Health Service Centre for Reviews and Dissemination: Revised inclusion criteria for DARE [DARE Web site]. October 16, 2000. Available at: http://agatha.york.ac.uk/dareinc.htm. Accessed June 18, 2002

National Health Service Centre for Reviews and Dissemination: Search strategies to identify reviews and meta-analyses in MEDLINE and CINAHL [NHS Centre for Reviews and Dissemination Web site]. April 2002. Available at: http://www.york.ac.uk/inst/crd/search.htm. Accessed September 5, 2002

National Health Service Information Authority: Information for health—1. An information strategy for the modern NHS [National Health Service Information Authority Web site]. July 24, 2001. Available at: http://www.nhsia.nhs.uk/def/pages/info4health/1.asp. Accessed June 18, 2002

Ovid: Databases@Ovid [Ovid products and services Web site]. 2002a. Available at: http://www.ovid.com/products/databases/index.cfm. Accessed June 19, 2002

Ovid: Evidence-based medicine reviews [Ovid products and services Web site]. 2002b. Available at: http://www.ovid.com/products/clinical/ebmr.cfm. Accessed June 19, 2002

Phillips B, Ball C, Sackett D, et al: Levels of evidence and grades of recommendations [Centre for Evidence-Based Medicine Web site]. May 2001. Available at http://www.cebm.net/levels_of_evidence.asp. Accessed June 27, 2003

Pittler MH, Ernst E: Efficacy of kava extract for treating anxiety: systematic review and meta-analysis. J Clin Psychopharmacol 20:84–89, 2000

Pittler MH, Ernst E: Kava extract for treating anxiety, in The Cochrane Library, Issue 2. Oxford, Update Software, 2002

Polmear A: Clinical evidence. ACP J Club 132:A15, 2000

Reeves BC, MacLehose RR, Harvey IM, et al: A review of observational, quasi-experimental and randomised study designs for the evaluation of the effectiveness of healthcare interventions, in The Advanced Handbook of Methods in Evidence Based Healthcare. Edited by Stevens A, Abrams K, Brazier J, et al. London, Sage, 2001, pp 116–135

Sackett DL, Strauss SE, Richardson WS, et al: Evidence-Based Medicine: How to Practice and Teach EBM, 2nd Edition. New York, Churchill Livingstone, 2000

Sensky T, Turkington D, Kingdon D, et al: A randomized controlled trial of cognitive-behavioral therapy for persistent symptoms in schizophrenia resistant to medication. Arch Gen Psychiatry 57:165–172, 2000

Shojania KG, Berg LA: Taking advantage of the explosion of systematic reviews: an efficient *MEDLINE* search strategy. Eff Clin Pract 4:157–162, 2001

Snowball R: Finding the evidence: an information skills approach, in Evidence-Based Practice: A Primer for Health Professionals. Edited by Dawes M, Davies P, Gray A, et al. New York, Churchill Livingstone, 1999, pp 15–46

University of Rochester Medical Center: Evidence-based filters for Ovid *CINAHL* [Edward G. Miner Library Web site]. 2002a. Available at: http://www.urmc.rochester.edu/Miner/Educ/ebnfilt.htm. Accessed June 27, 2003

University of Rochester Medical Center: Evidence-based filters for Ovid *MEDLINE* [Edward G. Miner Library Web site]. 2002b. Available at: http://www.urmc.rochester.edu/Miner/Educ/Expertsearch.html. Accessed June 19, 2002

Watson RJD, Richardson PH: Accessing the literature on outcome studies in group psychotherapy: the sensitivity and precision of *Medline* and *PsycINFO* bibliographic database searching. Br J Med Psychol 72:127–134, 1999

Watson RJD, Richardson PH: Identifying randomized controlled trials of cognitive therapy for depression: comparing the efficiency of *Embase, MEDLINE,* and *PsycINFO* bibliographic databases. Br J Med Psychol 72:535–542, 1999

Zaroukian MH: *PubMed* clinical queries: a web tool for filtered retrieval of citations relevant to evidence-based practice. ACP J Club 134:A15, 2001

5

CLINICAL TRIALS

After identifying one or more articles or other resources to answer a clinical question, the next step in the evidence-based medicine (EBM) process is to appraise the evidence. In this chapter and in Chapters 6–11, guidance on appraising a variety of different types of evidence is provided.

Because questions about therapy are among those most frequently asked by clinicians, we begin with a discussion of individual studies of therapies. Chapter 6 focuses on the appraisal of systematic reviews of therapies, whereas Chapter 7 focuses on the appraisal of treatment guidelines.

■ CONTROLLED VERSUS UNCONTROLLED STUDIES

Evidence about the effectiveness of a therapy can come from a variety of sources (Table 5–1). However, evidence from some types of studies is apt to be more biased and misleading than evidence from more rigorous study designs (Greenhalgh 2001; Guyatt 2002; Guyatt et al. 2002b; Lacchetti and Guyatt 2002), as explained below.

Single Case Reports

The least rigorous and potentially most biased type of evidence is that arising from a single case (Fletcher et al. 1996; Sackett et al. 1991). As clinicians, we like to believe that patients improve as a re-

TABLE 5–1.	**Types of studies used to address treatment effectiveness**

Uncontrolled studies

Single case reports

Case series

All-or-none case series[a]

Uncontrolled clinical trials

Controlled studies

Studies with historical controls

Studies with concurrent nonrandomized controls

    Patients of other physicians or clinical sites

    Patient or physician choice of treatment

    Systematic allocation

Randomized controlled trials[a]

With blinding[a]

Without blinding (open-label study)

[a]Strongest study designs.

sult of our efforts. We sometimes attribute patient improvement to a therapy when it was, in fact, the result of spontaneous improvement. Published single case reports have the added problem of publication bias: clinicians are more apt to report their successes with a novel treatment than they are their failures (Easterbrook et al. 1991; Fletcher et al. 1996; Montori and Guyatt 2002; Song et al. 2001). Although a single case report might result in a hypothesis that is later tested in a clinical trial, such reports cannot be relied on to guide treatment (Fletcher et al. 1996; Hennekens et al. 1987; Sackett et al. 1991).

Case Series

A case series is only slightly better than a single case report (Fletcher et al. 1996). Here the author is reporting on a series of patients treated for a particular condition. Because patients are not enrolled in a formal study, it is difficult to know whether the results reflect all patients being treated with a particular therapy or whether they reflect only the successes. As with single case reports, publication bias is a significant problem in case series, and they are best regarded as a source of ideas for further study.

A particular type of case series, though, does rank high in the evidence hierarchy: the "all-or-none" case series (Badenoch and Heneghan 2002) (Table 4–2, Chapter 4). An all-or-none case series refers to a series of patients who receive treatment for a disease with a universally bad (usually fatal) outcome. If a new treatment leads to a better outcome in all of the patients treated, there is strong evidence of treatment effectiveness. Examples of such an all-or-none case series are some of the earliest reports of the effectiveness of antibiotics in treating infections, which were performed 6 decades ago. It is difficult, however, to think of a psychiatric disorder for which an all-or-none case series would be an appropriate study design.

Uncontrolled Clinical Trials

An uncontrolled clinical trial is a step up from a case series. In this study design, patients enrolled in the study receive the new treatment, but there is no control group. Unlike in a case series, there is a study protocol in an uncontrolled clinical trial that specifies the nature of the subjects, treatment, and outcome measures. Because there is no control group, a variety of factors can bias the results. These factors include Hawthorne, experimenter expectancy (Pygmalion), and placebo effects; observer bias; regression toward the mean (Yudkin and Stratton 1996); and the natural history of the illness (Fletcher et al. 1996).

Historical Controls

Because improvement can occur spontaneously, as well as being a result of treatment, more convincing evidence about the effectiveness of a therapy comes from controlled trials. However, there are a variety of control groups that are sometimes used in clinical trials

(Altman 1991; Bland 2000; Fletcher et al. 1996). The first type is a historical control. In this situation, the outcomes of the patients receiving the experimental therapy in the trial are compared with the outcomes of patients with the same disorder and in the same treatment setting, but who have been treated in the past with another therapy. An example is the comparison of the lengths of stay of inpatients with schizophrenia treated with atypical antipsychotic medications versus those of inpatients with schizophrenia treated in the same institution a decade earlier, prior to the introduction of atypical antipsychotic medications. Although the use of historical controls might be convenient, the results can be biased by changes in diagnostic criteria, patient acuity and demographics, and other aspects of care that may have occurred over time (Fletcher et al. 1996; Hennekens et al. 1987). Furthermore, information about the historical control group typically comes from medical records recorded for purposes other than research, whereas the information about patients receiving the experimental therapy is collected with the purpose of the study in mind. This difference in the type of information collected is a form of observer bias (Daly and Bourke 2000). As a result, clinical trials using historical controls may often provide misleading answers and generally overestimate the true treatment effectiveness (Altman 1991; Bland 2000; Everitt 1989; Fletcher et al. 1996).

Nonrandomized Clinical Trials

There are also other types of nonrandomized clinical trials in which there are nonrandom assignments of subjects to one or more therapies (Altman 1991; Bland 2000; Fletcher et al. 1996). Examples include studies comparing treatments at one clinic versus treatments at another clinic or treatments by one set of providers versus treatments by another set of providers. Other examples include studies in which patients volunteer for the treatment they are to receive or in which they are systematically allocated to a treatment group (e.g., every other patient is assigned to a particular treatment). However, the key characteristic of such studies is that the subjects are not randomly assigned to the clinic, provider, or therapy. As a result, the various groups of subjects may differ at the outset of the study in ways that affect their prognosis, which is referred to as "selection bias" or "allocation bias" (Daly and Bourke 2000; Fletcher et al. 1996). Such studies are not true experiments, but are instead a type of observational study known as a *cohort study* (see Chapter 9).

Randomized Controlled Trials

The preferred study design to assess the effectiveness of a therapy is a randomized controlled trial (RCT) (Altman et al. 2001). In this study design, subjects are randomly assigned to either the control treatment or to one or more experimental treatments at the onset of the trial. Such randomization serves to make the control and experimental groups comparable in characteristics that may influence prognosis (confounding factors) (Altman 1991; Altman et al. 2001; Daly and Bourke 2000; Fletcher et al. 1996). In addition, conventional tests of statistical significance are all based on the assumption of random assignment of subjects (Altman 1991; Cummings et al. 2001; Daly and Bourke 2000). The blinding of subjects, clinicians, and raters is an additional attempt to reduce sources of bias in RCTs (see next section).

■ SOURCES OF BIAS

The clinician interested in a particular therapy wants an unbiased estimate of how it compares with another therapy or placebo. The results of a particular study may over- or underestimate the true difference in effectiveness of the two therapies. One reason for this is chance (random error), discussed further in the next section. The other reason is bias (defined as a systematic deviation from the true results), which results in either a systematic overestimation or a systematic underestimation of treatment effectiveness (Guyatt 2002; Sitthi-amorn and Poshyachinda 1993). One goal therefore in study design is to minimize bias (Altman 1991).

Confounding

One source of bias in a clinical trial is having experimental and control groups that differ at the onset of the study in characteristics that affect outcome (Guyatt 2002). This is a form of selection bias, and the subject characteristics that affect outcome are known as *confounding factors* (Altman et al. 2001; Daly and Bourke 2000; Jadad 1998). Confounding factors can include such variables as age, sex, ethnicity, illness severity, and comorbid illnesses. Adjustment for known confounding factors can occur in the statistical analysis of a study (Daly and Bourke 2000). Such statistical techniques cannot, however, adjust for unknown confounding factors. Randomization will, however, automatically adjust for such confounding factors by tending to make the treatment and control groups similar (Altman 1991; Altman et al. 2001; Daly and Bourke 2000; Fletcher et al. 1996; Guyatt 2002). Even with randomization, there will still be some differences between the experimental and control groups, but the statistical techniques that are used to analyze studies assume a certain amount of chance variation and take it into account (Daly and Bourke 2000). Indeed, if some form of matching is used to attempt to further minimize differences in known confounding factors between the experimental and control groups, this must be taken into account in the statistical analysis; if it is not, tests of statistical significance will be overly conservative (Daly and Bourke 2000; Peto et al. 1976).

Hawthorne Effect

There are also several nonspecific effects that can bias the results, including Hawthorne, Pygmalion, and placebo effects. The Hawthorne effect was first observed in studies of worker productivity at the Hawthorne Western Electric plant in Illinois in 1924 and refers to the tendency of subjects to do better solely because they are being studied (Fletcher et al. 1996; Holden 2001). Some of this may involve subject expectations, but it can also be the result of nonspecific effects of the study situation, such as the increased attention received. The Hawthorne effect is one reason why studies involving historical controls will produce biased results: experimental subjects know that they are part of a study and they therefore exhibit the Hawthorne effect, whereas historical controls were not originally experimental subjects and hence do not exhibit such an effect. The Hawthorne effect affects both the experimental and control groups in an RCT and thus is eliminated as a source of bias in this study design.

Pygmalion Effect and Cointerventions

The Pygmalion effect, also called the *experimenter expectancy effect*, was first described in educational research, in which it was demonstrated that teacher expectations affect pupil performance (Rosenthal and Jacobson 1968). Subsequent research has demonstrated that experimenter expectations regarding treatment effect may result in differential attention or interactions with some subjects, which results in a change in subject behavior in the direction of experimenter hypothesis (Rosenthal and Rosnow 1991). A related effect is that of a clinician involved in a trial providing additional care (e.g., time, support, etc.) to patients in one treatment group but not to those in the other treatment group. This effect is known as *cointervention* or *performance bias* (Altman et al. 2001; Fletcher et al. 1996; Guyatt 2002; Juni et al. 2001). In clinical trials, this effect can be minimized by blinding clinicians to the treatment being provided. Such blinding can occur in drug trials; however, such blinding is obviously impossible in trials of psychotherapy. It can, however, be minimized by documenting adherence to treatment protocols (Guyatt 2002).

Placebo Effect

The third nonspecific effect is the placebo effect (Crow et al. 2001; Kaptchuk 1998; Laporte and Figueras 1994). In this effect, it is the subject's expectation of improvement, combined with other nonspecific psychotherapeutic effects, that leads to improvement

(Chaput de Saintonge and Herxheimer 1994; Crow et al. 2001). The magnitude of the placebo response rate varies by disorder; it is greater in depression and anxiety disorders than in schizophrenia, but even in acute mania, there is a sizable placebo response (Charney et al. 2002) (Table 5–2). To separate the specific effects of a therapy from the nonspecific placebo effects, it is necessary to have a control group. Blinding the patient to the therapy being administered further reduces the placebo effect (Altman et al. 2001; Guyatt 2002), although this is far more difficult with psychosocial interventions than with drug therapies.

Observer, Detection, or Ascertainment Bias

The final important source of bias in a clinical trial is observer, detection, or ascertainment bias (Altman et al. 2001; Jadad 1998; Juni et al. 2001). If an interviewer or rater knows which treatment a patient is receiving, he or she may differentially inquire about certain symptoms or see improvement where none exists. Blinding the interviewer or rater to the treatment is an important way of minimizing observer bias (Altman et al. 2001; Guyatt 2002; Juni et al. 2001); however, it is difficult to do so entirely, because the treatment received may sometimes be discerned from treatment side effects or from a patient's comments.

Minimizing Bias Through Blinding

To minimize sources of bias, the optimal study design is an RCT in which the subjects, clinicians, and raters are all blind to the treatment being administered. This is possible in drug trials; however, in many trials involving psychosocial interventions, only the rater can be blinded. The terms *single blind*, *double blind*, and *triple blind* are often used to describe the design type of a study, but there is little agreement about the meaning of the terms (Devereaux et al. 2001; Montori et al. 2002). Consequently, it is preferable to simply specify which of the various participants in a study are blinded to the treatment (Altman et al. 2001; Devereaux et al. 2002; Fletcher et al. 1996).

TABLE 5–2. Placebo response rates in psychiatric disorders

Disorder	Outcome measure	Study duration	Placebo response rate (%)
Schizophrenia, acute episode	40% reduction in BPRS	6 weeks	8–32
Schizophrenia, maintenance	No relapse	9 months	34
Bipolar disorder, acute mania	50% reduction in Y-MRS	3 weeks	24
Bipolar disorder, maintenance	No relapse	2 years	19
Major depression	50% reduction in Ham-D	4–24 weeks (average 6 weeks)	30
Panic disorder	50% decrease in attacks	12 weeks	50
Social phobia	Much or very much improved	8–14 weeks	17–32
Obsessive-compulsive disorder	35% reduction in Y-BOCS	9–13 weeks	8–60

Note. BPRS=Brief Psychiatric Rating Scale; Ham-D=Hamilton Rating Scale for Depression; Y-BOCS=Yale-Brown Obsessive Compulsive Scale; Y-MRS=Young Mania Rating Scale.

Source. Data from Cookson et al. 2002; Walsh et al. 2002; Woods et al. 2001.

■ BASIC STATISTICAL CONCEPTS

In reviewing the results of a clinical trial, it is important to have at least a basic understanding of biostatistics. The following qualitative discussion does not discuss specific methods of statistical analysis or calculations; for such topics, the reader is referred to several excellent texts (Altman 1991; Bland 2000; Daly and Bourke 2000).

Hypothesis Testing

We begin with a hypothetical clinical trial comparing an experimental therapy with a control therapy. In this trial, participants are randomly assigned to one of two treatment groups. At the end of the trial, we assess the outcome in the two groups and find a difference. How do we know whether this difference is because the treatments differ in effectiveness or whether it is the result of chance? We know that even if the two treatments are identical, by chance alone there could be some difference in outcome. We therefore need to set a threshold, with differences in outcome greater than that threshold unlikely to be the result of chance alone. Conventionally, this threshold is set so that there is a 5% chance that a difference of that magnitude (or greater) will be the result of chance alone. In practice, an appropriate test statistic (e.g., t, F, or χ^2, etc.) is computed, from which a P value is derived. If $P < 0.05$, the difference is considered *statistically significant*. This approach to data analysis is referred to as *hypothesis testing*, in that a difference in treatment effect that exceeds a threshold leads us to reject the null hypothesis that there is no difference between treatments.

The results of this clinical trial can also be conceptualized as falling into one of four categories (Table 5–3). In reality, the experimental and control treatments are either equivalent or different. In our experiment, either the difference exceeds the preset threshold and is considered "statistically significant" or it does not. Let's now consider some of the various combinations.

TABLE 5–3. **Possible outcomes of a clinical trial**

| | True difference between treatments | |
Study outcome	No true difference	True difference exists
Difference found	False-positive result Type I error Probability=α	True-positive result Power=$1-\beta$
No difference found	True-negative result	False-negative result Type II error Probability=β

Type I Errors

If there is truly no difference between the experimental and control treatments, our experiment, by chance alone, might find a difference large enough to be called "statistically significant." This is the equivalent of a *false-positive* result on a diagnostic test. In statistical terms, it is considered a type I error. In the example above, the threshold has been set so that a type I error occurs <5% of the time. In statistical terms, it is represented as $\alpha=0.05$, where α is the probability of a type I error.

Type II Errors

Now suppose that there is truly a difference between the two treatments. In our experiment, sometimes we find a large difference between the treatment groups and sometimes, by chance alone, we may find only a small difference. Because we have set a threshold such that only differences that exceed the threshold are considered *statistically significant*, some of the results may not be considered *significant*, even though there is truly an underlying difference in the effectiveness of the two treatments. This is considered a type II error and is the equivalent of a *false-negative* result from a diagnostic test. The probability of a type II error occurring is represented by β.

Power

Ideally, we would like to have a high probability of detecting a difference when such a difference truly exists. This is the equivalent of a *true-positive* test result. Such a probability is given the term *power* and is represented by $1-\beta$.

The magnitude of the treatment effect needed for it to be considered *statistically significant* is determined by the variability of the results and by the number of subjects studied. The more variable the data, the larger the difference that must be obtained; the larger the number of subjects, the smaller the treatment difference needed for statistical significance. The same is true regarding the power of the experiment to detect a real treatment effect: the more variable the data, the larger the number of subjects required. In general, small studies often lack the power to detect clinically significant differences in treatment effectiveness; for that reason, such studies are considered by some to be unethical (Collins and MacMahon 2001; Halpern et al. 2002).

Confidence Intervals

The approach to data analysis that has been summarized thus far is the classical approach of *hypothesis testing,* in which a difference in treatment effect that exceeds a threshold is said to reject the null hypothesis that there is no difference between treatments. Such an approach focuses on *P* values and *statistical significance,* but it largely ignores the magnitude of any difference found (Sterne and Smith 2001).

An alternative approach that has become popular in recent years involves *confidence intervals* (CIs) (Gardner and Altman 2000). In this approach, the difference in treatment effectiveness between groups in the clinical trial is used to construct a CI. If a 95% CI is constructed, it implies that there is a 95% chance that the true difference in effectiveness lies within that interval. An interval that does not include zero is the equivalent of rejecting the null hypothesis (i.e., the equivalent of a "statistically significant" result).

There are several advantages to using CIs instead of hypothesis testing (Gardner and Altman 2000; Guyatt et al. 2002c). First, they provide a range in which the true treatment effectiveness is expected, with a narrow CI implying a precise estimate of treatment effectiveness. Second, in negative studies in which the null hypothesis is not rejected, CIs may suggest that a clinically important difference is present but that the power of the study to detect it was too low. There is a difference, for example, between a wide CI that barely overlaps zero and a narrow CI that centers on zero. In the first case, the width suggests that the study was too small to provide a precise estimate and that a large treatment difference cannot be excluded. In the second case, the estimate is quite precise and implies that any difference is too small to be clinically important. Finally, CIs are useful in systematic reviews and meta-analyses (see Chapter 6).

■ MEASURES OF TREATMENT EFFECTIVENESS

There are many different approaches for describing the effectiveness of a treatment (Jaeschke et al. 2002; Sackett et al. 1991). A drug company promoting a new medication may choose the measure that puts the drug in the best light. However, for a clinician choosing a therapy or advising a patient, there is a need for measures that accurately reflect how one treatment compares with either a placebo or another active treatment.

In psychiatric research, especially drug trials, investigators frequently use a variety of rating scales. In reporting the results of a study, they may compare the differences in rating scale scores of patients in the experimental and control groups. Although the use of such rating scales may be necessary for U.S. Food and Drug Administration (FDA) approval and may generate data that can be easily analyzed, they also have limitations. For example, clinicians and patients cannot easily appreciate the practical implications of a small difference on a particular scale.

In contrast, dichotomous outcome measures are more clinically useful than rating scales. Examples of such outcome measures include dying, being readmitted to the hospital, achieving full remission, being rated as "improved" or "much improved," or having at least a 50% decrease in score on a rating scale. These are all measures that most clinicians and patients consider clinically significant and that can be more readily understood than continuous rating scales that yield a numerical score. In addition, the use of such dichotomous outcome measures allows for the calculation of a number of useful measures of clinical importance. In illustrating these various measures and their calculation, we have used the results of a hypothetical RCT, comparing an antidepressant drug with a placebo for the treatment of major depression; the outcome measure was "remission" (see Table 5–4).

Percentage Response

In our hypothetical experiment, 60% of patients receiving the antidepressant drug responded. This is the simplest way of expressing the effectiveness of the antidepressant drug; however, it fails to take into account the high percentage of patients who responded to the placebo. To do so, a better measure of treatment response is thus necessary.

Relative Risk

In our example, 40% of patients receiving the placebo responded and 60% of patients receiving the placebo did not respond. By convention, when using relative risk (RR) as a measure of treatment effectiveness, results are expressed in terms of a bad outcome (e.g., nonresponse). An effective treatment is therefore one that reduces bad outcomes. Using this convention and our example, the percentage of control subjects *not* responding is called the *control event rate* (CER), which in this case is 60%.

For those receiving the antidepressant, 60% of patients responded, whereas 40% of patients did not respond. The percentage of experimental subjects *not* responding is called the *experimental event rate* (EER), which in this case is 40%.

TABLE 5–4. Results of hypothetical experiment used to illustrate measures of treatment effect size

Treatment	Not responding (%)	Responding (%)
Placebo	60	40
Antidepressant	40	60

Control event rate (CER)=60%
Experimental event rate (EER)=40%
Relative risk=EER/CER=40/60=0.67
Relative risk reduction=(CER−EER)/CER=20/60=0.33
Odds ratio=[EER/(1−EER)]/[CER(1−CER)]=[(40/60)/(60/40)]=0.44
Absolute risk reduction (ARR)=CER−EER=60%−40%=20%
Number needed to treat=1/ARR=1/(0.2)=5

The ratio of EER to CER is called *relative risk* (RR). In this case, RR=0.4/0.6=0.67, which means that patients receiving medication had only two-thirds the nonresponse rate of the placebo group. More effective treatments provide greater reductions in the risk of a negative outcome. RR values for effective treatments vary between 0 and 1, with smaller values indicating more effective treatments.

RR provides a comparison of the experimental and control treatments, but it can be misleading. For example, reducing the nonresponse rate from 90% to 45% yields the same RR as reducing it from 2% to 1%. In the first example, the treatment causes a much greater percentage of patients to respond than in the second example; however, both examples yield the same RR.

Relative Risk Reduction

Relative risk reduction (RRR) is calculated using the formulas RRR=(CER−EER)/CER or RRR=1−RR. Using the data in Table 5–4, RRR=0.2/0.6=0.33, which means that the nonresponse rate was decreased by one-third. Like RR, RRR varies between 0 and 1 for effective treatments; however, in this case, larger values (i.e., values closer to 1) indicate a more effective treatment. RRR has the same limitations as RR.

Odds Ratio

The odds ratio (OR) is a measure of treatment effect that is similar to RR. The odds of an event occurring are expressed as the ratio of the probability of the event occurring to the probability of the event not occurring. In our example, the odds of nonresponse are 1.5 (or 60 to 40) in the placebo group and 0.67 (or 40 to 60) in an experimental group. The OR is simply the ratio of the odds of a bad outcome in the experimental group divided by the odds of a bad outcome in a control group: 0.67/1.5=0.44. As with RR, for effective treatments, the OR varies between 0 and 1, smaller values being associated with a greater treatment effect. The OR is often used as an effect measure in meta-analyses because of its statistical properties (Deeks and Altman 2001).

Absolute Risk Reduction

Absolute risk reduction (ARR) is simply the difference between the CER and the EER. Using the data from Table 5–4, ARR=60%–40%=20%, which means that 20% fewer patients on medication failed to respond; conversely, 20% more patients on medication responded. Because this is an absolute (not relative) measure, it can be used to estimate the percentage of patients undergoing treatment who will benefit more from the experimental treatment than from the control treatment. ARR for effective treatments varies from 0% to 100% (or 0 and 1, if not expressed as a percentage), with larger values indicating more effective treatments. Unlike RR and RRR, ARR provides a measure of how many patients receiving treatment will benefit from it and thus avoids some of the limitations of these prior measures.

Number Needed to Treat

The measure believed by many to be the best expression of relative treatment effectiveness is number needed to treat (NNT) (Cook and Sackett 1995; Jaeschke et al. 2002; Laupacis et al. 1988; Sackett et al. 1991, 2000; Szatmari 1998). NNT is simply the reciprocal of the ARR. In our example, NNT=1/0.2=5, which means that for every five patients treated with medication, there will be one less case of nonresponse than if all patients had received the control treatment. Put another way, for every five patients treated with medication, there will be one additional patient who responds to medication who would not have responded to the placebo. The calculation of CIs for NNT is given by Altman (1998) and can be found in Appendix B.

NNT is believed by most clinical epidemiologists to be the least misleading and the most clinically useful measure of treatment effectiveness, although patients sometimes have difficulty understanding the concept (Kristiansen et al. 2002). Inclusion of NNT in the reporting of the results of clinical trials is recommended in the Consolidated Standards of Reporting Trials (CONSORT) guidelines (Altman et al. 2001). Despite this recommendation, relatively few trials report NNTs (Nuovo et al. 2002), so it is often necessary to go through the calculations yourself, using the data presented in a published article.

Examples of NNTs for common therapies for psychiatric disorders are given in Table 5–5. As can be seen, most psychiatric therapies have NNTs in the range of 3 to 6, which means that for every 3–6 patients treated, there is one good outcome that would not otherwise have occurred. For comparative purposes, in a 5-week follow-up of patients with acute myocardial infusion, using death as an outcome measure, streptokinase infusion had an NNT of 15; in a 5.5-year follow-up of patients with moderate hypertension (diastolic blood pressures of 90–109 mm Hg), using death, stroke, and myocardial infarction as outcomes, antihypertensive drugs had an NNT of 128 (Sackett et al. 2000). Hence, psychotropic medications are relatively effective when compared with other classes of drugs used in medicine.

■ CRITICAL APPRAISAL GUIDE FOR THERAPY STUDIES

This section of the chapter introduces a structured approach to the critical appraisal of therapy studies, which is mirrored in subsequent chapters that deal with other types of studies. The guidelines for appraisal of therapy studies are found in Table 5–6.

Is the Study Valid?

Before considering the results of a study, you must first focus on its "Methods" section to assess the study's validity. The first question to ask is whether the study was randomized with a concealed randomization list. Randomization minimizes bias that might result from patients with different prognoses being enrolled in either the

TABLE 5–5. Examples of numbers needed to treat (NNTs) for common psychiatric disorders and treatments

Disorder	Treatment comparison	Outcome measure	NNT
Major depression	Antidepressant vs. placebo	50% reduction in Ham-D	3
	IPT vs. clinical management	Recovery	5
	CBT plus antidepressant vs. monotherapy	50% reduction in Ham-D	5
Acute mania	Valproate or lithium vs. placebo	50% reduction in SADS-M	5
Bipolar disorder	Lithium vs. placebo	Relapse	3
Schizophrenia	Antipsychotic vs. placebo	40% reduction in BPRS or "much improved" CGI Scale	2–5
	Family intervention vs. usual care	Relapse	7
Panic disorder	SSRI vs. placebo	Panic free	3–6
Social phobia	Paroxetine vs. placebo	"Much improved" CGI Scale	3
	Group CBT vs. placebo	"Much improved" CGI Scale	3
Obsessive-compulsive disorder	SSRI vs. placebo	35% reduction in Y-BOCS	4–5
Bulimia nervosa	Antidepressants vs. placebo	Remission	9

Note. BPRS=Brief Psychiatric Rating Scale; CBT=cognitive behavioral therapy; CGI=Clinical Global Impression; Ham-D=Hamilton Rating Scale for Depression; IPT=interpersonal psychotherapy; SADS-M=Schizophrenia and Affective Disorders Scale, mania component; SSRI=selective serotonin reuptake inhibitor; Y-BOCS=Yale-Brown Obsessive Compulsive Scale.
Source. Data from Cookson et al. 2002; Geddes and Butler 2001; Hay and Bacaltchuk 2001; McIntosh and Lawrie 2001.

TABLE 5–6.　Critical appraisal guide for therapy studies

Is the study valid?

Is it a randomized controlled trial?

Was the randomization list concealed?

Were subjects and clinicians blinded to treatment being administered?

Were all subjects enrolled in the trial accounted for?

Were subjects analyzed in the groups to which they were assigned?

Despite randomization, were there clinically important differences
　between groups at the start of the trial?

Aside from the experimental treatment, were the groups treated equally?

Are the results important?

How large was the treatment effect (e.g., the number needed to treat)?

How precise were the results (e.g., the width of confidence intervals)?

Can I apply the results to my patient?

Is my patient too different from those in the study?

Is the treatment consistent with my patient's values and preferences?

Is the treatment feasible in my setting?

Source.　Adapted from Gray 2002; Guyatt et al. 2002a; Sackett et al. 2000.

---

experimental or control treatment group (Altman et al. 2001; Collins and MacMahon 2001; Fletcher et al. 1996; Lacchetti and Guyatt 2002; Juni et al. 2001; Sackett et al. 1991, 2000). Studies comparing randomized and nonrandomized trials of the same therapies have noted several instances of therapies that seemed effective in nonrandomized trials being much less effective or ineffective in randomized studies, although this is not always the case (Ioannidis et al. 2001; Kunz and Oxman 1998; Lacchetti and Guyatt 2002). Of equal importance, however, is that the allocation list is concealed. There have been some instances in which investigators have been able to determine the assignment of the next patient to be enrolled and have used that information to systematically enroll sicker patients into one treatment group (Altman and Schulz 2001). In addition, studies comparing trials in which allocation was concealed with those in which it was not concealed have found important differences in the size of the treatment effect (Altman and Schulz

2001; Juni et al. 2001; Kunz and Oxman 1998; Lacchetti and Guyatt 2002; Schulz 2000).

The next question to ask is whether subjects and clinicians were blinded to the treatment that was administered. As noted above, blinding represents an attempt to prevent observer bias, placebo effects, and experimenter expectancy effects from being responsible for any observed difference between the experimental and control groups. In general, nonblinded studies overestimate the true treatment effect size (Juni et al. 2001; Schulz 2000).

Third, you should check whether all subjects who entered the trial were accounted for at its conclusion and whether they were analyzed in the groups to which they had been randomized. Accounting for all subjects is made easier when a flow diagram of subject progress through the phases of a randomized trial is included in the paper, as suggested by the CONSORT guidelines (Altman et al. 2001; Moher et al. 2001). This is important because substantial loss of subjects to follow-up can seriously bias the results, an effect referred to as *attrition bias* (Guyatt and Devereaux 2002; Juni et al. 2001). It is sometimes stated that at least 80% follow-up is sufficient for the results to be valid (Streiner and Geddes 2001), although other authors argue that this rule of thumb is misleading (Guyatt et al. 2002a). Intent-to-treat analysis, which includes data on patients who did not complete the trial in their assigned group, is the preferred method of analyzing the data, although there are limitations to the method (Altman et al. 2001; Collins and MacMahon 2001; Guyatt and Devereaux 2002; Guyatt et al. 2002a; Juni et al. 2001; Streiner and Geddes 2001).

Finally, you should see if there are other differences between the control and experimental groups that could bias the results. For example, despite randomization, are there significant differences between the two groups at the start of the trial that could affect the outcome (i.e., confounding)? Aside from the experimental treatment, were the groups treated equally (i.e., no cointervention)?

Only after the validity has been appraised should you turn to the results. After all, if the results are not valid, it does not matter what they show.

Are the Results Important?

When reviewing the results of a study, it is necessary to give some thought to what you would consider a clinically significant outcome measurement. As noted above, these are often dichotomous outcome measures, and NNT should be calculated if it is not given in the results.

Can I Apply the Results to My Patient?

The final step in the appraisal process is to assess whether the results can be applied to your patient. Several considerations enter into this assessment. First, is your patient so different from the patients in the studies that the results do not apply? The question here can be reframed as: "Is the pathobiology of my patient so different from that of the study patients that the results cannot apply?" In general, the answer to this question is "no" (Sackett et al. 1991, 2000; Straus and McAlister 2001). There are, however, quantitative differences that may apply. In particular, if your patient's likelihood of improving *without* the experimental treatment is greater than that of patients in the study, then your patient will receive less benefit from the treatment than expected, based on the calculated NNT (Sackett et al. 2000). Methods of quantifying this are given by Sackett et al. (1991, 2000) and in Appendix B. Furukawa et al. (2002) have recently confirmed the validity of this approach.

Two additional questions must be asked before applying the treatment to your patient. The first is whether the treatment is consistent with your patient's values and preferences. The second is whether the treatment is feasible in your setting. Assuming that you have identified a valid study that has identified an effective treatment that can be applied to your patient, the next steps in the EBM process (Table 2–1, Chapter 2) are to apply the treatment and then to evaluate the outcome (see Chapter 12).

■ REFERENCES

Altman DG: Practical Statistics for Medical Research. Boca Raton, FL, Chapman and Hall, 1991

Altman DG: Confidence intervals for the number needed to treat. BMJ 317:1309–1312, 1998

Altman DG, Schulz KF: Statistics notes: concealing treatment allocation in randomised trials. BMJ 323:446–447, 2001

Altman DG, Schulz KF, Moher D, et al: The revised CONSORT statement for reporting randomized trials: explanation and elaboration. Ann Intern Med 134:663–694, 2001

Badenoch D, Heneghan C: Evidence-Based Medicine Toolkit. London, BMJ Books, 2002

Bland M: An Introduction to Medical Statistics, 3rd Edition. Oxford, UK, Oxford University Press, 2000

Chaput de Saintonge DM, Herxheimer A: Harnessing placebo effects in health care. Lancet 344:995–998, 1994

Charney DS, Nemeroff CB, Lewis L, et al: National Depressive and Manic-Depressive Association consensus statement on the use of placebo in clinical trials of mood disorders. Arch Gen Psychiatry 59:262–270, 2002

Collins R, MacMahon S: Reliable assessment of the effects of treatment on mortality and major morbidity, I: clinical trials. Lancet 357:373–380, 2001

Cook RJ, Sackett DL: The number needed to treat: a clinically useful measure of treatment effect. BMJ 310:452–454, 1995

Cookson J, Taylor D, Katona C: The Use of Drugs in Psychiatry: The Evidence from Psychopharmacology, 5th Edition. London, Gaskell, 2002

Crow R, Gage H, Hampson S, et al: The placebo effect: methodological process and implications of a structured review, in The Advanced Handbook of Methods in Evidence Based Healthcare. Edited by Stevens A, Abrams K, Brazier J, et al. London, Sage, 2001, pp 73–89

Cummings SR, Grady D, Hulley SB: Designing an experiment: clinical trials I, in Designing Clinical Research, 2nd Edition. Edited by Hulley SB, Cummings SR, Browner WS, et al. Philadelphia, PA, Lippincott Williams & Wilkins, 2001, pp 143–155

Daly LE, Bourke GJ: Interpretation and Uses of Medical Statistics, 5th Edition. Oxford, Blackwell Scientific, 2000

Deeks JJ, Altman DG: Effect measures for meta-analysis of trials with binary outcomes, in Systematic Reviews in Health Care: Meta-Analyses in Context, 2nd Edition. Edited by Egger M, Smith GD, Altman DG. London, BMJ Books, 2001, pp 313–335

Devereaux PJ, Manns BJ, Ghali WA, et al: Physician interpretations and textbook definitions of blinding terminology in randomized controlled trials. JAMA 285:2000–2003, 2001

Devereaux PJ, Bhandari M, Montori VM, et al: Double blind, you have been voted off the island! Evid Based Ment Health 5:36–37, 2002

Easterbrook PJ, Berlin JA, Gopalan R, et al: Publication bias in clinical research. Lancet 337:867–872, 1991

Everitt BS: Statistical Methods for Medical Investigations. New York, Oxford University Press, 1989

Fletcher RH, Fletcher SW, Wagner EH: Clinical Epidemiology: The Essentials, 3rd Edition. Baltimore, MD, Williams & Wilkins, 1996

Furukawa TA, Guyatt GA, Griffith LE: Can we individualize the 'number needed to treat'? An empirical study of summary effect measures in meta-analyses. Int J Epidemiol 31:72–76, 2002

Gardner MJ, Altman DG: Confidence intervals rather than P values, in Statistics With Confidence, 2nd Edition. Edited by Altman DG, Machin D, Bryant TN, et al. London, BMJ Books, 2000, pp 15–27

Geddes J, Butler R: Depressive disorders. Clinical Evidence 6:726–742, 2001

Gray GE: Evidence-based medicine: an introduction for psychiatrists. J Psychiatr Pract 8:5–13, 2002

Greenhalgh T: How to Read a Paper: The Basics of Evidence Based Medicine, 2nd Edition. London, BMJ Books, 2001

Guyatt G: Therapy and harm: why study results mislead—bias and random error, in Users' Guides to the Medical Literature: A Manual for Evidence-Based Clinical Practice. Edited by Guyatt G, Rennie D. Chicago, IL, AMA Press, 2002, pp 223–231

Guyatt G, Devereaux PJ: Therapy and validity: the principle of intention-to-treat, in Users' Guides to the Medical Literature: A Manual for Evidence-Based Clinical Practice. Edited by Guyatt G, Rennie D. Chicago, IL, AMA Press, 2002, pp 267–273

Guyatt G, Cook D, Devereaux PJ, et al: Therapy, in Users' Guides to the Medical Literature: A Manual for Evidence-Based Clinical Practice. Edited by Guyatt G, Rennie D. Chicago, IL, AMA Press, 2002a, pp 55–79

Guyatt G, Haynes B, Jaeschke R, et al: Introduction: the philosophy of evidence-based medicine, in Users' Guides to the Medical Literature: A Manual for Evidence-Based Clinical Practice. Edited by Guyatt G, Rennie D. Chicago, IL, AMA Press, 2002b, pp 3–12

Guyatt G, Walter S, Cook D, et al: Therapy and understanding the results: confidence intervals, in Users' Guides to the Medical Literature: A Manual for Evidence-Based Clinical Practice. Edited by Guyatt G, Rennie D. Chicago, IL, AMA Press, 2002c, pp 339–349

Halpern SD, Karlawish JHT, Berlin JA: The continuing unethical conduct of underpowered clinical trials. JAMA 288:358–362, 2002

Hay P, Bacaltchuk J: Bulimia nervosa. Clinical Evidence 6:715–725, 2001

Hennekens CH, Buring JE, Mayrent SL: Epidemiology in Medicine. Boston, MA, Little, Brown, 1987

Holden JD: Hawthorne effects and research into professional practice. J Eval Clin Pract 7:65–70, 2001

Ioannidis JPA, Haidich A-B, Pappa M, et al: Comparison of evidence of treatment effects in randomized and nonrandomized studies. JAMA 286:821–830, 2001

Jadad A: Randomised Controlled Trials. London, BMJ Books, 1998

Jaeschke R, Guyatt G, Barratt A: Therapy and understanding the results: measures of association, in Users' Guides to the Medical Literature: A Manual for Evidence-Based Clinical Practice. Edited by Guyatt G, Rennie D. Chicago, IL, AMA Press, 2002, pp 351–368

Juni P, Altman DG, Egger M: Assessing the quality of controlled clinical trials. BMJ 323:42–26, 2001

Kaptchuk TJ: Powerful placebo: the dark side of the randomised clinical trial. Lancet 351:1722–1725, 1998

Kristiansen IS, Gyrd-Hansen D, Nexoe J, et al: Number needed to treat: easily understood and intuitively meaningful? Theoretical considerations and a randomized trial. J Clin Epidemiol 55:888–892, 2002

Kunz R, Oxman AD: The unpredictability paradox: review of empirical comparisons of randomised and non-randomised clinical trials. BMJ 317:1185–1190, 1998

Lacchetti C, Guyatt G: Therapy and validity: surprising results of randomized controlled trials, in Users' Guides to the Medical Literature: A Manual for Evidence-Based Clinical Practice. Edited by Guyatt G, Rennie D. Chicago, IL, AMA Press, 2002, pp 247–265

Laporte J-R, Figueras A: Placebo effects in psychiatry. Lancet 344:1206–1209, 1994

Laupacis A, Sackett DL, Roberts RS: An assessment of clinically useful measures of the consequences of treatment. N Engl J Med 318:1728–1733, 1988

McIntosh A, Lawrie S: Schizophrenia. Clinical Evidence 6:776–797, 2001

Moher D, Schulz KF, Altman D: The CONSORT statement: revised recommendation for improving the quality of reports of parallel-group randomized trials. JAMA 285:1987–1991, 2001

Montori V, Guyatt G: Summarizing the evidence: publication bias, in Users' Guides to the Medical Literature: A Manual for Evidence-Based Clinical Practice. Edited by Guyatt G, Rennie D. Chicago, IL, AMA Press, 2002, pp 529–538

Montori VM, Bhandari M, Devereaux PJ, et al: In the dark: the reporting of blinding status in randomized controlled trials. J Clin Epidemiol 55:787–790, 2002

Nuovo J, Melnikow J, Chang D: Reporting number needed to treat and absolute risk reduction in randomized controlled trials. JAMA 287:2813–2814, 2002

Peto R, Pike MC, Armitage P, et al: Design and analysis of randomized clinical trials requiring prolonged observation of each patient, I: introduction and design. Br J Cancer 34:585–612, 1976

Rosenthal R, Jacobson L: Pygmalion in the Classroom. New York, Holt, Rinehart and Winston, 1968

Rosenthal R, Rosnow RL: Essentials of Behavioral Research: Methods and Data Analysis, 2nd Edition. Boston, MA, McGraw-Hill, 1991

Sackett DL, Haynes RB, Guyatt GH, et al: Clinical Epidemiology: A Basic Science for Clinical Medicine, 2nd Edition. Boston, MA, Little, Brown, 1991

Sackett DL, Strauss SE, Richardson WS, et al: Evidence-Based Medicine: How to Practice and Teach EBM, 2nd Edition. New York, Churchill Livingstone, 2000

Schulz KF: Assessing allocation concealment and blinding in randomised controlled trials: why bother? Evid Based Ment Health 3:4–5, 2000

Sitthi-amorn C, Poshyachinda V: Bias. Lancet 342:286–288, 1993

Song F, Eastwood A, Gilbody S, et al: Publication and related biases, in The Advanced Handbook of Methods in Evidence Based Healthcare. Edited by Stevens A, Abrams K, Brazier J, et al. London, Sage, 2001, pp 371–390

Sterne JAC, Smith GD: Sifting the evidence: what's wrong with significance tests? BMJ 322:226–231, 2001

Straus SE, McAlister F: Applying the results of trials and systematic reviews to our individual patients. Evid Based Ment Health 4:6–7, 2001

Streiner D, Geddes J: Intention to treat analysis in clinical trials when there are missing data. Evid Based Ment Health 4:70–71, 2001

Szatmari P: Some useful concepts and terms used in articles about treatment. Evid Based Ment Health 1:39–40, 1998

Walsh BT, Seidman SN, Sysko R, et al: Placebo response in studies of major depression: variable, substantial, and growing. JAMA 287:1840–1847, 2002

Woods SW, Stolar M, Sernyak MJ, et al: Consistency of atypical antipsychotic superiority to placebo in recent clinical trials. Biol Psychiatry 49:64–70, 2001

Yudkin PL, Stratton IM: How to deal with regression to the mean in intervention studies. Lancet 347:241–243, 1996

6

SYSTEMATIC REVIEWS
AND META-ANALYSES

Chapter 5 discussed individual studies of therapies. As was pointed out in that chapter, both false-positive and false-negative results can occur in clinical trials because of chance and bias. In particular, false negatives are common because studies are often too small to detect important treatment effects. As a result, when attempting to answer a clinical question, it is best not to depend on the results of a single clinical trial. It is preferable instead to "average out" the results of all such clinical trials related to a specific clinical question because this will give a better estimate of the treatment effect than the results of any single study. This is exactly what is done in a meta-analysis, and it is why systematic reviews rank at the top of the evidence hierarchy (Table 4–2, Chapter 4).

■ NARRATIVE REVIEWS VERSUS
SYSTEMATIC REVIEWS

In the typical *journalistic* or *narrative* review article, the author attempts to present a coherent review of a topic, selectively citing the literature to support the statement made in the article. When studies of a treatment are not in agreement, the author of the review may tally the positive and negative results (sometimes called *vote counting*), indicating that controversy exists and that more research is needed to resolve the issue.

Although such reviews are common in medical journals

(Rochon et al. 2002), they are often misleading, reflecting the author's biases in selectively reviewing the literature (Cook et al. 1998; Egger et al. 2001c; Greenhalgh 2001). Such reviews may contribute to delays in implementing changes in clinical practice that are based on important research findings (Egger et al. 2001c).

The systematic review is a better alternative to the traditional review (Cook et al. 1998; Egger et al. 2001c; Greenhalgh 2001). Such a review focuses on a specific clinical question, involves a comprehensive literature search, and often combines the study results mathematically through meta-analytic techniques (Cook et al. 1998).

■ CONDUCTING A SYSTEMATIC REVIEW

The steps involved in conducting a systematic review are summarized in Table 6–1 and are described briefly below. Readers who want more detail about the conduct of systematic reviews are referred to several recent textbooks (Clarke and Oxman 2002; Egger et al. 2001b; Glasziou et al. 2001; National Health Service Centre for Reviews and Dissemination 2001; Petitti 2000).

Formulate the Question

The first step in the process is formulating the question. The process is similar to that of the evidence-based medicine (EBM) model (Chapter 3) and involves a similar 4-part PICO question (patient/problem, intervention, comparison, and outcome).

Locate Studies

The second step in the process involves finding all of the relevant studies. Such a search involves using the usual online databases described in Chapter 4, but using filters for *sensitivity* (rather than for *specificity*) (Glasziou et al. 2001; Robinson and Dickersin 2002). Such a strategy will, however, miss many early (pre-1990) studies, non–English language studies, and unpublished studies, so addi-

TABLE 6–1.	Steps in conducting a systematic review

1. Formulate the question

2. Locate studies
   Online databases (e.g., *MEDLINE, EMBASE*, etc.)
   Registers of clinical trials
       Cochrane Controlled Trial Registry
       *meta*Register
   Contact authors or manufacturers
   Check reference lists
   Perform manual searches

3. Assess study quality
   Rating scales
   Two or more reviewers

4. Extract and summarize the data
   Tables
   Forest plots
   Pooled effect size and confidence intervals

tional effort may be needed to identify such studies (Egger and Smith 1998; Egger et al. 2001a; Glasziou et al. 2001; Lefebvre and Clarke 2001). Methods that authors undertake to identify such studies include contacting authors of published studies or manufacturers of drugs, checking reference lists of published studies or prior reviews ("snowballing"), manually searching journals or proceeding abstracts that are not abstracted in MEDLINE or similar databases, and checking databases of clinical trials (Glasziou et al. 2001; Helmer et al. 2001; Lefebvre and Clarke 2001). The latter includes the Cochrane Controlled Trials Registry (available as part of Ovid's *EBM Reviews* database) and the *meta*Register of Controlled Trials (http://www.controlled-trials.com). If such measures are not taken, several sources of bias may influence the results of the review, including publication bias and language bias (Table 6–2).

Publication bias, also known as the *file drawer problem*, refers to a tendency to preferentially publish "positive" results (Egger

TABLE 6–2. **Types of reporting bias in systematic reviews**

Type of bias	Description
Publication bias	Results are more apt to be published if they are significant.
Time lag bias	Significant results are published sooner than nonsignificant results.
Language bias	Significant results are submitted to English-language journals, nonsignificant results to non–English language journals.
Database bias	Studies with significant results are more likely to be published in a journal that is indexed in a database.
Citation bias	Likelihood of article being cited depends on results.
Duplicate publication bias	Results of study appear in more than one publication.
Outcome reporting bias	Selective reporting of some study results.

Source.   Adapted from Egger and Smith 1998; Egger et al. 2001a.

and Smith 1998; Egger et al. 2001a; Montori and Guyatt 2002; Montori et al. 2000; Rosenthal 1979; Sterne et al. 2001). Although it is clear that publication bias occurs, the reasons for it are a topic of some debate, but they include decisions by the investigators, journal editors and reviewers, and pharmaceutical company influences (Egger and Smith 1998; Egger et al. 2001a; Montori and Guyatt 2002; Montori et al. 2000; Olson et al. 2002; Song et al. 2001; Stern and Simes 1997; Thornton and Lee 2000).

Language bias can occur if English-language journals publish a greater proportion of positive studies than do non–English language journals. Such a bias could occur if foreign investigators preferentially submit positive findings to English-language journals (Egger and Smith 1998; Egger et al. 2001a; Song et al. 2001). *Location bias*, a similar type of bias, refers to the tendency to publish lower-quality positive studies of complementary medicine in low-impact journals (Pittler et al. 2000). The extent to which language and location bias occurs seems to vary, depending on the medical specialty and the disease in question (Juni et al. 2002; Moher et al. 2000).

Assess Study Quality

Because the goal of the search strategy is to be as inclusive as possible to avoid missing relevant studies, a search will typically identify a large number of studies, many of which are either irrelevant or of poor quality. Including such irrelevant or poor-quality studies in the review and subsequent meta-analysis yields misleading results. Statisticians refer to this as "garbage in, garbage out."

As was discussed in Chapter 5, evidence from less rigorously designed studies is more apt to be biased and misleading than is evidence from more rigorously designed studies (Greenhalgh 2001; Guyatt 2002; Lacchetti and Guyatt 2002; Schulz et al. 1995). It is therefore necessary to appraise the studies identified in the search and to limit further analysis to those studies that meet certain quality criteria (Juni et al. 2001). The method of doing so is similar to the approach used in Chapter 5 to appraise a randomized controlled trial (RCT). A standardized approach to appraisal, generally involving two reviewers, should be used to avoid biasing the review (Glasziou et al. 2001; Moher et al. 2001). A variety of instruments for rating the quality of studies have been developed for this purpose, but there is no single best instrument (Juni et al. 2001; West et al. 2002).

Specific study quality aspects may have a greater impact on estimates of treatment effect than others, but this depends on the particular disease and treatment in question (Balk et al. 2002). Nonrandomized trials, trials with inadequate allocation concealment, and unblinded trials tend to overestimate the magnitude of a treatment's effectiveness, although this is not uniformly true for all diseases and their treatments (Altman and Schulz 2001; Ioannidis et al. 2001; Juni et al. 2001; Kjaergard et al. 2001; Kunz and Oxman 1998; Lacchetti and Guyatt 2002; Schulz 2000). As a general rule, though, selecting higher-quality studies will lead to a less biased—and generally less optimistic—view of a treatment's effectiveness.

In the process of appraising study quality, an attempt should also be made to identify duplicate or overlapping publications. This can occur, for example, if preliminary data are first published, followed by a second (more complete) publication. It can also occur if different outcome measures are each presented in a separate publication. If such duplicate or overlapping publications are not identified, the same study may be overrepresented in any meta-analysis, a result known as *multiple publication bias* (Egger and Smith 1998; Tramer et al. 1997).

Extract and Summarize the Data

Once studies meeting the quality criteria are identified, data are abstracted. Such data include methodological details regarding the study population, intervention, outcome measures, and so forth, as well as study results. Such data are typically presented in tabular form in the review, and numerical results are often displayed graphically and combined in a meta-analysis. A list of studies that were identified, appraised, and excluded from the review is generally included in the review, along with the reasons for exclusion.

Time and Effort Involved in Systematic Reviews

The process described above is conceptually simple; however, it is obviously quite time-consuming, especially if the literature search identifies a large number of studies that must then be assessed for quality. Allen and Olkin (1999) found that systematic review requires 200–2,500 man-hours of effort (median, 1,110 hours). About one-half of this effort is spent on the search and retrieval process.

A systematic review is generally a group effort because of the considerable effort involved in its production. Two international collaborative efforts that are involved in producing systematic reviews are the Cochrane Collaboration and the Campbell Collaboration (Antes and Oxman 2001; Cochrane Collaboration 1997; Davies and Boruch 2001). Table 4–5 in Chapter 4 lists some of the other organizations involved in producing systematic reviews.

■ META-ANALYSIS

Meta-analysis refers to the statistical integration of the results of several independent studies (Egger and Smith 1997). This section provides a short nonmathematical overview of meta-analysis. Readers who want an in-depth discussion are referred to several excellent recent texts (Egger et al. 2001b; Petitti 2000; Sutton et al. 2000).

Meta-analysis involves more than "vote-tallying" or merely taking a simple average of the results of various studies. Instead, meta-analysis gives more weight to large studies than to small studies, because the results of small studies are subject to more random variability (see Chapter 5). The specific methods by which this is accomplished depend on whether the outcome variable is dichotomous or continuous.

Dichotomous Outcome Measures

As was discussed in Chapter 5, dichotomous outcome measures, such as dying, being readmitted to the hospital, achieving full remission, being rated as "improved" or "much improved," or having at least a 50% decrease in score on a rating scale, are often among the most clinically useful and readily understandable measures. Dichotomous measures are also favored in systematic reviews because of the ease of combining the data in meta-analyses.

Odds Ratio

The measure of treatment effect that is most commonly used in systematic reviews and meta-analyses is the odds ratio (OR). Calculation of the OR was described in Chapter 5. By convention, the outcome measures used in meta-analysis are adverse outcomes; therefore, effective treatments have ORs <1.0.

The reason that the OR is so frequently used in meta-analyses is that there are several straightforward methods of combining ORs from multiple studies (Deeks et al. 2001; Petitti 2000; Sutton et al. 2000). The two most common methods are the Mantel-Haenszel method (Mantel-Haenszel 1959) and the Peto method (Yusuf et al. 1985). Both methods involve producing a weighted average OR, with larger trials (which have narrower confidence intervals [CIs] for their ORs) being given greater weight than smaller trials (with wider CIs for their ORs), although they differ in the exact weighting used. Both methods assume a "fixed effects" model (see next section). The DerSimonian and Laird method (DerSimonian and Laird 1986), used under the "random effects" model, gives somewhat more weight to smaller studies and produces a wider CI for the pooled OR estimate than do the other two methods.

The drawback of using the OR as a measure of treatment effectiveness is that it is not as easily interpretable as relative risk (RR) or number needed to treat (NNT) (Deeks and Altman 2001). Although the OR approximates RR when the frequency of rare outcomes is low (<10%), the two measures diverge as the outcome frequency increases, with the OR overestimating RR (Egger et al. 1997a). Under such circumstances, misinterpretation of an OR as RR will lead the reader to overestimate or underestimate the effects of a treatment (Deeks and Altman 2001).

Number Needed to Treat

Although NNT is believed by many to be the best expression of relative treatment effectiveness (Cook and Sackett 1995; Sackett et al. 1991, 2000), its mathematical properties are such that it cannot be directly used in a meta-analysis (Deeks and Altman 2001). NNT can, however, be calculated from the summary OR and the estimated control event rate (CER), using the formula in Appendix B. This approach assumes that the OR for a particular treatment comparison is independent of the CER. Empirically, this appears to be the case (Furukawa et al. 2002; McAlister 2002).

Continuous Outcome Measures

Continuous outcome measures, which include such things as body weight, intelligence quotient, or scores on a rating scale, are common in psychiatric research. In meta-analyses of continuous outcome measures, standardized mean differences, not the means of the outcome measures, are used as the measure of treatment effect (Deeks et al. 2001; Petitti 2000; Sutton et al. 2000). The results of each study are transformed into a standardized mean difference (represented by the letter d), using the following formula:

$$d = \frac{(\text{mean}_e - \text{mean}_c)}{\text{SD}_p}$$

where mean_e and mean_c are the means for the experimental and control groups, respectively, and SD_p is the pooled estimate of the standard deviation (SD) of the outcome measure. The results are then pooled by taking a weighted average of the d's for each study, with the weight for a given study being the inverse of the variance of that study's effect size (Deeks et al. 2001; Petitti 2000; Sutton et al. 2000).

The standardized mean difference is a measure of the degree of overlap of the experimental and control group results, expressed in terms of standard deviations (Freemantle and Geddes 1998). If

$d=0$, the means of the control and experimental groups are identical. If $d=1$, the mean of the experimental group is 1 SD above the mean of the control group. From a standard statistical table for a normal distribution, this is equivalent to saying that 84% of the control group has scores below the mean of the experimental group. A table for interpreting the standardized mean difference is given in Appendix B.

Fixed and Random Effects Models

As noted above, there are both "fixed effects" and "random effects" models for combining the results of clinical trials. The choice of model is a topic of debate among statisticians, and readers are referred elsewhere for a more complete discussion (Egger et al. 2001b; Freemantle and Geddes 1998; Montori et al. 2002; Petitti 2000; Sutton et al. 2000). At the risk of oversimplifying a complex issue, it is probably sufficient to say that fixed effects models assume that there is no heterogeneity in study results, whereas random effects models assume that there is heterogeneity. As a result, the random effects model should be preferred when heterogeneity is present.

If there is no heterogeneity, both models will produce similar pooled estimates of the OR, but the confidence intervals obtained using the random effects models are wider (less precise). As a result, the null hypothesis (i.e., that there is no difference between the two treatments) will be rejected less often if calculations are performed using the random effects model. This has led to the claim that the random effects model is overly conservative when there is minimal heterogeneity. In contrast, when there is heterogeneity, hypothesis testing, using the random effects model, gives the more appropriate results. (See Chapter 5 for further discussion of hypothesis testing.)

A second practical consideration is that the random effects model gives more equal weighting to large and small studies than does the fixed effect model, which gives more weight to large studies. If there is heterogeneity between the results of large and small studies as the result of either publication bias or differences in quality that varies by study size, the pooled estimate obtained with the random effects model will be more subject to such biases than the estimate obtained with the fixed effects model.

As a practical note, in most cases the two models give similar results. When the results differ, there is generally heterogeneity present, and the causes for the heterogeneity need to be taken into account rather than only relying on the pooled estimate of treatment effect.

Forest Plots

Many systematic reviews present their results graphically, in the form of *forest plots* (Egger and Smith 2001; Egger et al. 1997a; Glasziou et al. 2001; Lewis and Clarke 2001; Sutton et al. 2000), also referred to as a *blobbograms* (Freemantle and Geddes 1998). An example of a forest plot is given in Figure 6–1. In this example, the results of each individual study are given by a horizontal bar, with the width of the bar representing the 95% CI for the OR in that study. For each study, a black diamond is used to represent the OR; the size of the diamond is a measure of the size of the study (and hence the weight given to it). Unshaded diamonds are used to indicate the pooled OR, with the width of the diamond indicating the 95% confidence interval for the pooled estimate.

Heterogeneity

Heterogeneity is present when the results from individual studies differ by more than what was expected by chance alone (Freemantle and Geddes 1998; Sutton et al. 2000). Heterogeneity can be assessed either informally (graphically) or through statistical techniques (Sutton et al. 2000).

The informal graphical approach uses forest plots. If there is considerable overlap between the CI bars for the various studies, there is no heterogeneity. Conversely, if the CI bars for some studies do not overlap those of other studies, heterogeneity is present. Fig-

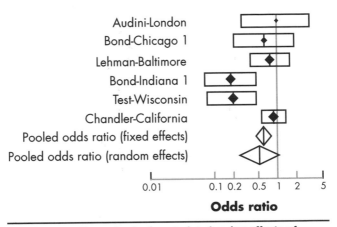

FIGURE 6–1. **Example of a forest plot showing effects of assertive community treatment versus usual care on odds of hospitalization of patients with severe mental illness.**

Source. Reprinted from Freemantle N, Geddes J: "Understanding and Interpreting Systematic Reviews and Meta-Analyses, II: Meta-Analyses." *Evidence-Based Mental Health* 1:102–104, 1998. Copyright 1998 BMJ Publishing Group. Used with permission.

ure 6–1 shows that four of the studies found no treatment effect, whereas two studies found the experimental treatment to be significantly better than the control treatment. It can also be seen that the CIs of the four *negative* studies overlap each other and that the CIs of the two *positive* studies also overlap each other. However, the bars for the *positive* studies do not overlap the Chandler-California study at all; in addition, they barely overlap the Lehman-Baltimore study. Thus, there is heterogeneity in the study results.

The formal statistical approach is to use a chi-square test for heterogeneity. This involves the calculation of a statistic, "Q," which has a chi-square distribution with 1 degree of freedom less than the number of studies. Details of the calculations are given elsewhere (Deeks et al. 2001; Petitti 2000; Sutton et al. 2000).

As noted above, when heterogeneity is detected, the random effects model gives a better estimate of pooled effect size than the fixed effects model. However, the analysis should not stop there. Instead, an attempt should be made to assess the cause of the heterogeneity (Deeks et al. 2001; Glasziou et al. 2001; Petitti 2000; Sutton et al. 2000; Thompson 1994, 2001). Some of the causes of heterogeneity include differences between studies in patient population (e.g., disease severity or other prognostic factors), nature of the intervention (e.g., medication dose, frequency or number of psychotherapy sessions, or presence of cointerventions), compliance, outcome measures, study duration, study quality, and other sources of bias (Glasziou et al. 2001; Sutton et al. 2000).

If the source of the heterogeneity can be identified, it is sometimes useful to present the results by subgroup (Sutton et al. 2000). Unfortunately, differences in subgroups identified in this *post hoc* fashion may represent the effects of chance or bias rather than true differences in response to treatment (Smith and Egger 2001; Sutton et al. 2000). If, however, such subgroup differences are anticipated from the start of the meta-analysis process (i.e., prior to looking at the forest plot, combining the results, or testing for heterogeneity), then such subgroup analyses may be appropriate.

Funnel Plots and Publication Bias

As previously noted, publication bias is often a concern in systematic reviews. Furthermore, it can bias the results of a meta-analysis, especially if the random effects model is assumed.

Publication bias is usually assessed with a *funnel plot* (Egger et al. 1997b; Glasziou et al. 2001; Montori et al. 2000; Montori and Guyatt 2002; Sterne et al. 2001). In a funnel plot, the x axis is treatment effect and the y axis is either study size or a measure of the study standard error, with standard error now considered the preferable measure (Sterne and Egger 2001).

Examples of funnel plots are given in Figure 6–2. Figure 6–2A

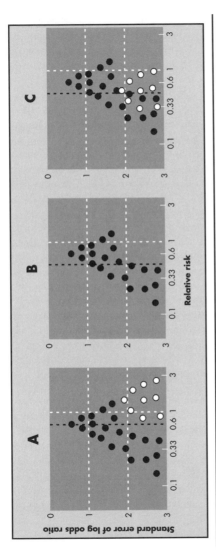

FIGURE 6–2. Examples of funnel plots.

(A) Symmetrical funnel plot demonstrating that results from all studies are centered around common relative risk but those from small studies vary more from the mean than do those from large studies.

(B) Publication bias occurs when small negative studies (shown as open circles in [A]) are not published. This results in the asymmetrical funnel plot shown in (B).

(C) Smaller studies are often of lower methodological quality, producing biased results (open circles). This can also produce an asymmetrical funnel plot.

Source. Reprinted from Sterne JAC, Egger M, Smith GD: "Investigating and Dealing With Publication and Other Biases in Meta-Analysis." *British Medical Journal* 323:101–105, 2001. Copyright 2001 BMJ Publishing Group. Used with permission.

shows a situation in which there is no publication bias. It can be seen that the plot is symmetrical. On average, the results of smaller studies are the same as those of larger studies; however, results from small studies are more variable. As a result, they deviate more from the mean, producing the funnel shape.

If there is publication bias, there will be a tendency to publish *positive* small study results, but not *negative* small study results. Such a tendency diminishes as the size of the study increases. In Figure 6–2A, the open circles represent the "negative" studies; these studies were not published. Removing these studies gives the asymmetrical funnel plot in Figure 6–2B.

Because small studies may be of lower methodological quality, they may be more likely to exaggerate the effects of a treatment (Kjaergard et al. 2001; Sterne et al. 2000, 2001). This situation, too, can produce an asymmetrical funnel plot, as demonstrated in Figure 6–2C.

Sensitivity Analysis

Questions often arise about whether a particular study or set of studies should be included or not in a meta-analysis because of differences in study design (e.g., patient population, treatment, cointervention, outcome measure, duration, quality). In sensitivity analysis, the calculations are performed with and without a particular subset of studies to see whether this has any effect on the overall results (Egger and Smith 2001; Sutton 2000).

A good example of the usefulness of sensitivity analysis comes from a systematic review of the effectiveness of antidepressants versus placebo in dysthymic disorder (Lima and Moncrieff 2002). Because the pre-1980 literature does not use the term *dysthymic disorder*, patients with this disorder were labeled as having *depressive neurosis*, *neurotic depression*, *depressive personality disorder*, and so forth. Lima and Moncrieff included studies of such patients but then used sensitivity analysis to demonstrate that the results were the same if the diagnosis was limited to *dysthymia* as they would be if these other studies were included.

■ CRITICAL APPRAISAL GUIDE FOR SYSTEMATIC REVIEWS

Even systematic reviews from respected sources can have methodological problems (Hopayian 2001; Olsen et al. 2001); therefore, all such reviews should be appraised by the reader. Several guides have been developed for the critical appraisal of systematic reviews (Badenoch and Heneghan 2002; Centre for Evidence-Based Medicine n.d.; Centre for Evidence-Based Mental Health n.d.; Freemantle and Geddes 1998; Geddes et al. 1998; Greenhalgh 2001; Oxman et al. 2002; Sackett et al. 2000; Seers 1999; Shea et al. 2001). One such guide appears in Table 6–3.

Did the Review Address a Clearly Defined Issue?

The first step in planning a systematic review is formulating the question. The authors of the review should indicate the 4-part PICO question (Chapter 3) that they are trying to address. Unless the question itself is clear, it is likely that the subsequent literature search will be unfocused. As a result, if the clinical question is not clear, you should probably try to find another review (Seers 1999). However, a review also may be either too broad or too narrow (Oxman et al. 2002). For example, a systematic review of psychotherapy for mental illness is such a broad topic that it is unlikely that the reviewers could do it justice within the confines of even a book-length review. Conversely, a systematic review of a topic that is too narrow may not generate appropriate studies, and such a review may be of limited generalizability.

Did the Authors Select the Right Sort of Studies?

As noted in Table 4–1 in Chapter 4, some study designs are better than others for answering particular types of clinical questions. For example, as was discussed in Chapter 5, the RCT is the preferred study design for answering therapy questions. The authors of a review should specify their inclusion criteria for which types of stud-

---

TABLE 6–3. **Critical appraisal guide for systematic reviews**

Did the review address a clearly defined issue?

Is the 4-part PICO question clearly identified?

Is the topic too broad or too narrow?

Did the authors select the right types of studies?

Are the inclusion criteria specified?

Do the authors specify the appropriate type of study to answer the question?

Were all relevant studies included?

How comprehensive was the search strategy?

Were appropriate electronic databases used?

Did the databases include non–English-language journals?

Did the authors go beyond electronic databases (e.g., personal contacts, manual searches, etc.)?

Was the quality of the studies addressed?

Were explicit criteria used?

Were two raters used, with a procedure for resolving differences?

Are the results similar from study to study? If not, was heterogeneity addressed?

Are the results clearly displayed (e.g., in a forest plot)?

Is there evidence of heterogeneity?

Are the reasons for the differences in study results discussed?

What are the overall results (with confidence intervals)?

What is the pooled effect measure, with confidence intervals?

Does it indicate that the two treatments are significantly different?

Can I apply the results to my patient?

Is my patient too different from those in the study?

What is the number needed to treat for my patient?

Is the treatment consistent with my patient's values and preferences?

Is the treatment feasible in my setting?

Note. PICO=patient/problem, intervention, comparison, outcome.

Source. Adapted from Centre for Evidence-Based Mental Health n.d.; Greenhalgh 2001; Oxman et al. 2002; Sackett et al. 2000; Seers 1999.

ies were selected, and these criteria should be appropriate to the clinical question being asked (Seers 1999).

Were All Relevant Studies Included?

Several questions can be asked with regard to the studies included. How comprehensive was the search strategy? Did the authors only search *MEDLINE* or did they also search other online databases? Did the authors make other attempts to locate studies—for example, did they contact authors of published studies or manufacturers of drugs, check reference lists of published studies or prior reviews (i.e., snowballing), perform manual searches of journals or proceeding abstracts that are not abstracted in *MEDLINE* or similar databases, and check databases of clinical trials? If such measures are not taken, several sources of bias could influence the results, including publication bias and language bias (Table 6–2).

Was the Quality of the Studies Addressed?

As was discussed above and in Chapter 5, evidence from less rigorously designed studies is more apt to be biased and misleading than is evidence from more rigorously designed studies. The authors of the review should describe the criteria used for assessing quality, including the minimum quality needed for inclusion. For example, they may decide to include only RCTs with at least 80% follow-up and intention-to-treat analysis. Whatever the criteria, they should be explicit and decided in advance so that they are not influenced by study results (Silagy et al. 2002). In addition, the assessment of quality should generally involve two reviewers and a mechanism for resolving a difference between them (Glasziou et al. 2001; Oxman et al. 2002; Seers 1999). Reviews should list which studies were excluded from the analysis for quality reasons, and the reason for exclusion should be given.

Are the Results Similar From Study to Study?

Many systematic reviews present their results graphically in the form of forest plots. As previously discussed, forest plots can be used to assess whether the results are similar from study to study. The more formal statistical approach is to use a chi-square test for heterogeneity.

If heterogeneity is detected, an attempt should be made to assess the cause of the heterogeneity. Subgroup analysis may be appropriate if the rationale was identified beforehand. Sensitivity analysis may also indicate whether the inclusion of certain studies has a significant impact on the pooled measure of treatment effect.

What Are the Overall Results (With Confidence Intervals)?

The results of a meta-analysis will generally be presented as a forest diagram that includes a pooled effect measure and its confidence intervals. For dichotomous outcome measures, this is an OR; for continuous measures, it is a standardized mean difference. If the confidence intervals for the pooled OR include 1 or if the confidence intervals for the standardized mean difference include 0, there is no statistically significant difference between the experimental and control treatments.

Can I Apply the Results to My Patient?

The final step in the appraisal process is to assess whether the results can be applied to your patient. As with the discussion of a single therapy study in Chapter 5, several considerations enter into this assessment.

First, is your patient so different from those in the studies that the results do not apply? The question can again be reframed in the following way: "Is the pathobiology of my patient so different from that of the study patients that the results cannot apply?" Typically, the answer to this question is "no," although there may be quantitative differences. To quantify the likelihood of your patient benefiting from a treatment, it is first necessary to convert the pooled estimate of the OR to NNT (McQuay and Moore 1998; Sackett et al. 2000) (see Appendix B).

Finally, there are two additional questions that must be considered before applying the treatment to your patient. First, is the treatment consistent with your patient's values and preferences? Second, is the treatment feasible in your setting? Assuming that you have identified a high-quality systematic review that has identified an effective treatment for your patient, the next steps in the EBM process (Table 2–1, Chapter 2) are to treat the patient and to evaluate the outcome (see Chapter 12).

■ REFERENCES

Allen IE, Olkin I: Estimating time to conduct a meta-analysis from number of citations retrieved. JAMA 2892:634–635, 1999

Altman DG, Schulz KF: Statistics notes: concealing treatment allocation in randomised trials. BMJ 323:446–447, 2001

Antes G, Oxman AD: The Cochrane Collaboration in the 20th century, in Systematic Reviews in Health Care: Meta-Analysis in Context. Edited by Egger M, Smith GD, Altman DG. London, BMJ Books, 2001, pp 447–458

Badenoch D, Heneghan C: Evidence-Based Medicine Toolkit. London, BMJ Books, 2002

Balk EM, Bonis PAL, Moskowitz H, et al: Correlation of quality measures with estimates of treatment effect in meta-analyses of randomized controlled trials. JAMA 287:2973–2982, 2002

Centre for Evidence-Based Medicine: Critical Appraisal Worksheet for Systematic Review of Therapy [Centre for Evidence-Based Medicine Web site]. n.d. Available at: http://www.cemb.net/worksheet—overview.asp. Accessed June 28, 2003

Centre for Evidence-Based Mental Health: Critical appraisal form for an overview [Centre for Evidence-Based Mental Health Web site]. n.d. Available at: http://cebmh.warne.ox.ac.uk/cebmh/education/appraisal/index.html. Accessed September 9, 2002

Clarke M, Oxman AD (eds): Cochrane reviewers' handbook 4.1.6. [Cochrane Collaboration Web site]. April 2002. Available at: http://www.cochrane.dk/cochrane/handbook/handbook.htm. Accessed September 5, 2002

Cochrane Collaboration: The Cochrane Collaboration leaflet [Cochrane Collaboration Web site]. Available at: http://www.cochrane.org/cochrane/leaflet.htm. September 1997. Accessed June 18, 2002

Cook DJ, Mulrow CD, Haynes RB: Synthesis of best evidence for clinical decisions, in Systematic Reviews: Synthesis of Best Evidence for Health Care Decisions. Edited by Mulrow C, Cook D. Philadelphia, PA, American College of Physicians, 1998, pp 5–12

Cook RJ, Sackett DL: The number needed to treat: a clinically useful measure of treatment effect. BMJ 310:452–454, 1995

Davies P, Boruch R: The Campbell Collaboration does for public policy what Cochrane does for public health. BMJ 323:294–295, 2001

Deeks JJ, Altman DG: Effect measures for meta-analyses of trials with binary outcomes, in Systematic Reviews in Health Care. Edited by Egger M, Smith GD, Altman DG. London, BMJ Books, 2001, pp 313–335

Deeks JJ, Altman DG, Bradburn MJ: Statistical methods for examining heterogeneity and combining results from several studies in meta-analysis, in Systematic Reviews in Health Care. Edited by Egger M, Smith GD, Altman DG. London, BMJ Books, 2001, pp 285–312

DerSimonian R, Laird N: Meta-analysis in clinical trials. Control Clin Trials 7:177–188, 1986

Egger M, Smith GD: Meta-analysis: potentials and promise. BMJ 315:1371–1374, 1997

Egger M, Smith GD: Bias in location and selection of studies. BMJ 316:61–66, 1998

Egger M, Smith GD: Principles and procedures for systematic reviews, in Systematic Reviews in Health Care. Edited by Egger M, Smith GD, Altman DG. London, BMJ Books, 2001, pp 23–42

Egger M, Smith GD, Phillips AN: Meta-analysis: principles and procedures. BMJ 315:1533–1537, 1997a

Egger M, Smith GD, Schneider M, et al: Bias in meta-analysis detected by a simple, graphical test. BMJ 315:629–634, 1997b

Egger M, Dickersin K, Smith GD: Problems and limitations in conducting systematic reviews, in Systematic Reviews in Health Care. Edited by Egger M, Smith GD, Altman DG. London, BMJ Books, 2001a, pp 43–68

Egger M, Smith GD, Altman DG (eds): Systematic Reviews in Health Care. London, BMJ Books, 2001b

Egger M, Smith GD, O'Rourke K: Rationale, potentials, and promise of systematic reviews, in Systematic Reviews in Health Care. Edited by Egger M, Smith GD, Altman DG. London, BMJ Books, 2001c, pp 3–19

Freemantle N, Geddes J: Understanding and interpreting reviews and meta-analyses, II: meta-analyses. Evid Based Ment Health 1:102–104, 1998

Furukawa TA, Guyatt GH, Griffith LE: Can we individualize the 'number needed to treat'? An empirical study of summary effect measures in meta-analysis. Int J Epidemiol 31:72–76, 2002

Geddes J, Freemantle N, Streiner D, et al: Understanding and interpreting reviews and meta-analyses, I: rationale, search strategy, and describing results. Evid Based Ment Health 1:68–69, 1998

Glasziou P, Irwig L, Bain C, et al (eds): Systematic Reviews in Health Care: A Practical Guide. New York, Cambridge University Press, 2001

Greenhalgh T: How to Read a Paper: The Basics of Evidence Based Medicine, 2nd Edition. London, BMJ Books, 2001

Guyatt G: Therapy and harm: why study results mislead—bias and random error, in Users' Guides to the Medical Literature: A Manual for Evidence-Based Clinical Practice. Edited by Guyatt G, Rennie D. Chicago, IL, AMA Press, 2002, pp 223–231

Helmer D, Savoie I, Green C, et al: Evidence-based practice: extending the search to find material for the systematic review. Bull Med Libr Assoc 89:346–352, 2001

Hopayian K: The need for caution in interpreting high quality systematic reviews. BMJ 323:681–684, 2001

Ioannidis JPA, Haidich A-B, Pappa M, et al: Comparison of evidence of treatment effects in randomized and nonrandomized studies. JAMA 286:821–830, 2001

Juni P, Altman DG, Egger M: Assessing the quality of randomised controlled trials, in Systematic Reviews in Health Care. Edited by Egger M, Smith GD, Altman DG. London, BMJ Books, 2001, pp 87–108

Juni P, Holenstein F, Sterne J, et al: Direction and impact of language bias in meta-analyses of controlled trials: empirical study. Int J Epidemiol 31:115–123, 2002

Kjaergard LL, Villumsen J, Gluud C: Reported methodologic quality and discrepancies between large and small randomized trials in meta-analyses. Ann Intern Med 135:982–989, 2001

Kunz R, Oxman AD: The unpredictability paradox: review of empirical comparisons of randomised and non-randomised clinical trials. BMJ 317:1185–1190, 1998

Lacchetti C, Guyatt G: Therapy and validity: surprising results of randomized controlled trials, in Users' Guides to the Medical Literature: A Manual for Evidence-Based Clinical Practice. Edited by Guyatt G, Rennie D. Chicago, IL, AMA Press, 2002, pp 247–265

Lefebvre C, Clarke MJ: Identifying randomised trials, in Systematic Reviews in Health Care. Edited by Egger M, Smith GD, Altman DG. London, BMJ Books, 2001, pp 69–86

Lewis S, Clarke M: Forest plots: trying to see the wood and the trees. BMJ 322:1479–80, 2001

Lima MS, Moncrieff S: Drugs versus placebo for dysthymia, in The Cochrane Library, Issue 3. Oxford, Update Software, 2002.

Mantel N, Haenszel W: Statistical aspects of the analysis of data from retrospective studies of disease. J Natl Cancer Inst 22:719–748, 1959

McAlister FA: Commentary: relative treatment effects are consistent across the spectrum of underlying risks…usually. Int J Epidemiol 31:76–77, 2002

McQuay HJ, Moore RA: Using numerical results from systematic reviews in clinical practice, in Systematic Reviews: Synthesis of Best Evidence for Health Care Decisions. Edited by Mulrow C, Cook D. Philadelphia, PA, American College of Physicians, 1998, pp 23–36

Moher D, Klassen TP, Schulz KF, et al: What contributions do languages other than English make on the results of meta-analyses? J Clin Epidemiol 5:964–972, 2000

Moher D, Klassen TP, Jones AL, et al: Assessing the quality of reports of randomised trials included in meta-analyses: attitudes, practice, evidence and guides, in The Advanced Handbook of Methods in Evidence Based Healthcare. Edited by Stevens A, Abrams K, Brazier J, et al. London, Sage, 2001, pp 409–425

Montori V, Guyatt G: Summarizing the evidence: publication bias, in Users' Guides to the Medical Literature: A Manual for Evidence-Based Clinical Practice. Edited by Guyatt G, Rennie D. Chicago, IL, AMA Press, 2002, pp 529–538

Montori VM, Smieja M, Guyatt GH: Publication bias: a brief review for clinicians. Mayo Clin Proc 75:1284–1288, 2000

Montori V, Guyatt G, Oxman A, et al: Summarizing the evidence: fixed-effects and random-effects models, in Users' Guides to the Medical Literature: A Manual for Evidence-Based Clinical Practice. Edited by Guyatt G, Rennie D. Chicago, IL, AMA Press, 2002, pp 539–545

National Health Service Centre for Reviews and Dissemination [NHS CRD]: Undertaking systematic reviews of research on effectiveness, CRD Report No 4, 2nd Edition [NHS CRD Web site]. March 2001. Available at: http://www.york.ac.uk/inst/crd/report4.htm. Accessed September 5, 2002

Olsen O, Middleton P, Ezzo J, et al: Quality of Cochrane reviews: assessment of sample from 1998. BMJ 323:829–832, 2001

Olson CM, Rennie D, Cook D, et al: Publication bias in editorial decision making. JAMA 287:2825–2828, 2002

Oxman A, Guyatt G, Cook D, et al: Summarizing the evidence, in Users' Guides to the Medical Literature: A Manual for Evidence-Based Clinical Practice. Edited by Guyatt G, Rennie D. Chicago, IL, AMA Press, 2002, pp 155–173

Petitti DB: Meta-Analysis, Decision Analysis, and Cost-Effectiveness Analysis: Methods for Quantitative Synthesis in Medicine, 2nd Edition. New York, Oxford University Press, 2000

Pittler MH, Abbot NC, Harkness EF, et al: Location bias in controlled clinical trials of complementary/alternative therapies. J Clin Epidemiol 53:485–489, 2000

Robinson KA, Dickersin K: Development of a highly sensitive search strategy for the retrieval of reports of controlled trials using PubMed. Int J Epidemiol 31:150–153, 2002

Rochon PA, Bero LA, Bay AM, et al: Comparison of review articles published in peer-reviewed and throwaway journals. JAMA 287:2853–2856, 2002

Rosenthal R: The 'file drawer problem' and tolerance for null results. Psychol Bull 86:638–641, 1979

Sackett DL, Haynes RB, Guyatt GH, et al: Clinical Epidemiology: A Basic Science for Clinical Medicine, 2nd Edition. Boston, Little, Brown, 1991

Sackett DL, Strauss SE, Richardson WS, et al: Evidence-Based Medicine: How to Practice and Teach EBM, 2nd Edition. New York, Churchill Livingstone, 2000

Schulz KF: Assessing allocation concealment and blinding in randomised controlled trials: why bother? Evid Based Ment Health 3:4–5, 2000

Schulz KF, Chalmers I, Hayes RJ, et al: Empirical evidence of bias: dimensions of methodological quality associated with estimates of treatment effects in controlled trials. JAMA 273:408–412, 1995

Seers K: Systematic review, in Evidence-Based Medicine: A Primer for Health Care Professionals. Edited by Dawes M, Davies P, Gray A, et al. Edinburgh, Churchill-Livingstone, 1999, pp 85–100

Shea B, Dube C, Moher D: Assessing the quality of reports of systematic reviews: the QUORUM statement compared to other tools, in Systematic Reviews in Health Care. Edited by Egger M, Smith GD, Altman DG. London, BMJ Books, 2001, pp 122–139

Silagy CA, Middleton P, Hopewell S: Publishing protocols of systematic reviews: comparing what was done to what was planned. JAMA 287: 2831–2834, 2002

Smith GD, Egger M: Going beyond the grand mean: subgroup analysis in meta-analysis of randomised trials, in Systematic Reviews in Health Care. Edited by Egger M, Smith GD, Altman DG. London, BMJ Books, 2001, pp 143–156

Song F, Eastwood A, Gilbody S, et al: Publication and related biases, in The Advanced Handbook of Methods in Evidence Based Healthcare. Edited by Stevens A, Abrams K, Brazier J, et al. London, Sage, 2001, pp 371–390

Stern JM, Simes RJ: Publication bias: evidence of delayed publication in a cohort study of clinical research projects. BMJ 315:640–645, 1997

Sterne JAC, Egger M: Funnel plots for detecting bias in meta-analysis: guidelines on choice of axis. J Clin Epidemiol 54:1046–1055, 2001

Sterne JAC, Gavaghan D, Egger M: Publication and related bias in meta-analysis: power of statistical tests and prevalence in the literature. J Clin Epidemiol 53:1119–1129, 2000

Sterne JAC, Egger M, Smith GD: Investigating and dealing with publication and other biases in meta-analysis. BMJ 323:101–105, 2001

Sutton AJ, Abrams KR, Jones DR, et al: Methods for Meta-Analysis in Medical Research. New York, Wiley, 2000

Thompson SG: Why sources of heterogeneity in meta-analysis should be investigated. BMJ 309:1351–1355, 1994

Thompson SG: Why and how sources of heterogeneity should be investigated, in Systematic Reviews in Health Care. Edited by Egger M, Smith GD, Altman DG. London, BMJ Books, 2001, pp 157–175

Thornton A, Lee P: Publication bias in meta-analysis: its causes and consequences. J Clin Epidemiol 53:207–216, 2000

Tramer MR, Reynolds DJM, Moore RA, et al: Impact of covert duplicate publication on meta-analysis: a case study. BMJ 315:635–640, 1997

West S, King V, Carey TS, et al: Systems to Rate the Strength of Scientific Evidence. Evidence Report/Technology Assessment, No 47. Rockville, MD, Agency for Healthcare Research and Quality, 2002

Yusuf S, Peto R, Lewis J, et al: Beta blockade during and after myocardial infarction: an overview of the randomized trials. Prog Cardiovasc Dis 27:335–371, 1985

7

CLINICAL PRACTICE GUIDELINES

Clinical practice guidelines are generally defined as "systematically developed statements to assist practitioner decisions about appropriate health care for specific clinical circumstances" (Field and Lohr 1990, p 1). Over the past two decades, there has been considerable interest and activity in developing these guidelines for a variety of clinical conditions, driven by concerns about variability in clinical practice, cost, quality, and legal liability (Birkmeyer 2001; Field and Lohr 1992; Greenhalgh 2001; Woolf et al. 1999a).

■ ROLE OF GUIDELINES IN EVIDENCE-BASED PRACTICE

Most clinical practice guidelines represent an attempt to improve clinical care by focusing on effective evidence-based interventions. Although practice guidelines are sometimes equated with evidence-based medicine (EBM) (Grol 2001a), they should be viewed as distinct for several reasons (Gray 2002; Lipman 2000). First, as noted below, not all practice guidelines are based on the best evidence, as derived from a systematic review of the medical literature (Browman 2001; Drake et al. 2001; Gray 2002; Greenhalgh 2001; Kahn et al. 1997; Woolf et al. 1999a). All guidelines involve some degree of judgment and bias in their development (Browman 2001; Drake et al. 2001; Greenhalgh 2001), the extent of which is often unstated. In addition, clinical practice guidelines are often introduced as part of a "top-down" approach to changing clinician behavior, leading to clinician resistance (Haines and Jones 1994; Lipman 2000). In contrast, EBM, as described in Chapters 1 and 2, represents a "bottom-up" approach in which clinicians make decisions based on ability to search and appraise the medical literature.

Evidence-based clinical practice guidelines, however, can play a role in the EBM process as an information resource (Grimshaw and Eccles 2001; Woolf et al. 1999a) (see Chapter 4). Studies of practicing clinicians have found that clinicians often do not have the time to search and appraise the literature themselves, but that they would welcome evidence-based guidelines when faced with clinical questions (McColl et al. 1998; Young and Ward 2001). In such cases, high-quality evidence-based guidelines can provide useful guidance (Feder et al. 1999; Grimshaw and Eccles 2001; Woolf et al. 1999). In addition, such evidence-based guidelines generally either include or reference a systematic review of the relevant literature.

■ SOURCES OF GUIDELINES

Clinical practice guidelines have been developed by a variety of organizations and now number in the thousands (Woolf et al. 1999a, 1999b). Some of the guidelines are evidence based; others are not. As described in Chapter 4, a useful starting point in searching for evidence-based clinical practice guidelines is the National Guideline Clearinghouse (http://www.guideline.gov).

American Psychiatric Association

The evidence-based guidelines most familiar to American psychiatrists are the ones developed by the American Psychiatric Association (APA). These guidelines currently cover the major psychiatric disorders and are available both in print form (APA 2002) and online (http://www.psych.org/clin_res/prac_guide.cfm). The APA guidelines are based on a systematic review of treatment options, with the use of expert opinion to synthesize the findings. One advantage of the APA guidelines is that they include a useful review of the relevant literature.

Agency for Healthcare Research and Quality

The Agency for Healthcare Research and Quality (AHRQ) and its predecessor, the Agency for Health Care Policy and Research (AHCPR), have also developed evidence-based practice guidelines for depression (Agency for Health Care Policy and Research 1993a, 1993b) and schizophrenia (Lehman and Steinwachs 1998). As with the APA guidelines, these guidelines are based on a rigorous systematic review of the literature. Unlike in the APA guidelines, there is no mechanism for updating the recommendations, and the depression guideline is considerably out of date (Shekelle et al. 2001).

Expert Opinion

Unlike the APA, AHCPR, and AHRQ guidelines, the Expert Consensus Guidelines (2002) are not based on an extensive review of the literature. Instead, they are based on expert opinion (Frances et al. 1998), and therefore they cannot be considered evidence-based guidelines (Kahn et al. 1997). There are numerous instances in which expert opinion on the treatment of medical conditions has been proved wrong by well-conducted research (Antman et al. 1992; Greenhalgh 2001; Mulrow 1994; Sackett et al. 1991); therefore, opinion does not necessarily provide the best guide to clinical practice. However, expert opinion can play a role in situations in which there simply is no evidence from well-conducted clinical trials.

Texas Medication Algorithms

The Texas Medication Algorithm Project (TMAP) is an attempt to provide prescribing guidelines for use within the Texas public mental health system (TMAP 2002). There are currently algorithms for schizophrenia, depression, and bipolar disorder (Texas Implementation of Medication Algorithms 2002). As with the Expert Consensus Guidelines (2002), the TMAP algorithms are based largely on expert consensus and cannot be considered to be evidence based (Gilbert et al. 1998).

Other Organizations

A variety of other organizations, such as the Canadian Medical Association, New Zealand Guidelines Group, Scottish Intercollegiate Guidelines Network, and U.K. National Health Service (NHS), have produced high-quality evidence-based clinical practice guidelines (see Chapter 4).

■ DIFFERENCES AMONG GUIDELINES

As indicated in the above section, not all guidelines are based on the best available evidence. Some guidelines are based on expert consensus and are not truly evidence based (Berg et al. 1997; Browman 2001). Guidelines also differ considerably in comprehensiveness, format, frequency of review, and ease of use. Milner and Valenstein (2002) have provided a useful comparison of several of the guidelines for the treatment of schizophrenia that details many of these differences. Those produced by the APA, AHRQ, and the other organizations listed in Table 4–4 in Chapter 4 are generally of high quality, but any guideline should be assessed prior to its use (see below).

■ DEVELOPING EVIDENCE-BASED
PRACTICE GUIDELINES

The development of evidence-based clinical practice guidelines is generally viewed as a 6-step process (Eccles et al. 2001; Shekelle et al. 1999a, 1999b) (Table 7–1).

Identify the Topic

The first step in the guideline development process is to identify and refine the subject of the guideline. Given the large number of diagnoses and the time needed to develop guidelines, some prioritiza-

TABLE 7–1.	Steps in developing evidence-based practice guidelines

1. Identify and refine the topic of the guideline

2. Convene an appropriate group
Typically 6–20 members
Requires both clinical and statistical expertise
Should be multidisciplinary

3. Gather and assess the evidence
Systematic review of literature
Hierarchy of evidence

4. Translate the evidence into recommendations
Some degree of clinical judgment always needed a) to weigh conflicting information and b) when there is little evidence

5. Use outside reviewers to review the recommendations
Should include users, as well as experts
Assess for validity and practicality

6. Update the guideline periodically

Source. Adapted from Berg et al. 1997; Eccles et al. 2001; Shekelle et al. 1999a.

tion must occur. Often this step is based on considerations such as the prevalence or economic impact of a disorder (Berg et al. 1997; Cook et al. 1998; Shekelle et al. 1999a, 1999b). Furthermore, decisions must be made on the scope of the guideline (e.g., whether it should be restricted to pharmacological treatment or whether it should include psychosocial interventions, patient education, etc.). Some authors suggest creating a "causal pathway" that diagrams the links between steps in a diagnostic or treatment process and the potential outcomes (benefits or harms) that could occur (Berg et al. 1997; Shekelle et al. 1999a, 1999b).

Convene a Group

The group convened to develop the guideline should include individuals with expertise in statistics and epidemiology, as well as clinical expertise related to the condition or treatment that will be the topic of the guideline (Berg et al. 1997; Shekelle et al. 1999a, 1999b). Such groups typically have 6–20 members, with one member serving as the group leader to moderate discussions, often supported by a project management team (Shekelle et al. 1999a, 1999b). It is best to convene a multidisciplinary group that includes representation from all of the stakeholders involved in implementing the guideline (Cook et al. 1998; Shekelle et al. 1999a, 1999b). Concerns have recently been raised regarding the extent to which pharmaceutical company relationships may influence decisions by members of guideline development groups (Choudhry et al. 2002; Greenhalgh 2001).

Gather and Assess the Evidence

The third step is to gather and assess the evidence regarding the subject of the guideline. Preexisting systematic reviews can be helpful in this step, provided that the systematic reviews themselves are valid (Browman 2001; Cook et al. 1998; Eccles et al. 2001; Shekelle et al. 1999a, 1999b). If they are not, then the guideline development group must develop its own systematic review (see Chapter 6).

In the process of assessing the evidence, different weight must be given to evidence from different study designs. As described in Chapter 4, hierarchies of evidence have been developed for this process (Badenoch and Heneghan 2002; Harbour and Miller 2001; Shekelle et al. 1999a, 1999b).

Translate the Evidence Into Recommendations

The fourth step is to translate the evidence into the recommendations that will make up the guideline. Clinical judgment is required in this step, both to weigh conflicting information and to make recommendations when there is little or no hard evidence (Harbour and Miller 2001; Shekelle et al. 1999a, 1999b). A variety of procedures have been developed to facilitate this process (Black et al. 2001; Kahn et al. 1997). Final recommendations should include an indication of the strength of evidence on which they are based (Harbour and Miller 2001; Pinsky and Deyo 2000; Shekelle et al. 1999a, 1999b).

Obtain Outside Review

The fifth step in the guideline development process is external review to ensure that the guidelines are both valid and practical. This step should be done by potential users of the guidelines, as well as those with clinical and scientific expertise (Berg et al. 1997; Shekelle et al. 1999a, 1999b).

Update Guidelines Periodically

It is recognized that guidelines may become outdated as new diagnostic and treatment procedures are developed and as additional knowledge is acquired regarding the benefits and harms of existing procedures. Based on a review of published AHRQ guidelines, Shekelle et al. (2001) suggested that guidelines should be assessed for validity every 3 years, although the generalizability of this recommendation to other guidelines remains in doubt (Browman 2001). In any case, some strategy must exist for periodically evaluating new evidence and for updating guidelines as necessary (Browman 2001; Shekelle et al. 1999a, 1999b, 2001).

■ CRITICAL APPRAISAL OF GUIDELINES

Because of the variable nature of the guideline development process, with some guidelines linked more closely to the research evidence than others, it is necessary to critically appraise guidelines before following their recommendations (Feder et al. 1999). Several guidelines have been developed for the critical appraisal of clinical practice guidelines (Greenhalgh 2001; Grimshaw and Eccles 2001; Guyatt et al. 2002; Pinsky and Deyo 2000; Sackett et al. 2000; Snowball 1999). Table 7–2 presents one approach.

Is the Guideline Valid?

The first part of the appraisal concerns the validity of the clinical practice guidelines.

TABLE 7–2.	Critical appraisal guide for a clinical practice guideline

Is the guideline valid?

Did the developers carry out a systematic review of the literature?

Were all relevant treatment options and outcomes considered?

Did the developers specify and make explicit the values associated with various outcomes?

Did the developers indicate the level of evidence (and sources) upon which each recommendation was based?

Is the guideline applicable to my practice?

Is the burden of illness too low to warrant implementation?

Are the beliefs of my patients incompatible with the guidelines?

Are the costs and other barriers of implementation too high?

Source. Adapted from Greenhalgh 2001; Guyatt et al. 2002; Sackett et al. 2000.

Did the Developers Carry Out a Systematic Review?

The development of a systematic review is what distinguishes evidence-based guidelines from opinion-based guidelines.

Were All Relevant Treatment Options and Outcomes Considered?

There are several questions that should be asked with regard to treatment options and outcome. For example, do the guidelines only mention pharmacotherapy, or do they include psychotherapy and other psychosocial interventions? Have the developers considered potential harms from the interventions, or have they only considered the benefits? It is more likely that these issues will be addressed if the group developing the guidelines is multidisciplinary rather than one limited by narrow expertise (Guyatt et al. 2002).

Did the Developers Specify Values Associated With Various Outcomes?

Reasonable people can make very different recommendations based on the same evidence, depending on the value attached to different outcomes. In a review of atypical antipsychotics in the treatment of schizophrenia, Geddes et al. (2000) concluded that atypical and conventional antipsychotics were equal in effectiveness and tolerability. The authors then went on to recommend conventional antipsychotics as first-line drugs because of cost considerations. Using the same data, Kapur and Remington (2000), reached the opposite conclusion, giving more value to the differences in risk of extrapyramidal side effects and less value to other side effects and to economic considerations. In weighing benefits and risks, guideline developers should be clear as to how they arrive at a particular recommendation (Guyatt et al. 2002).

Did the Developers Indicate the Level of Evidence and Sources Upon Which Each Recommendation Was Based?

If guideline developers indicate the level of evidence and sources upon which each recommendation is based, the user can determine which recommendations are based on strong evidence and which recommendations are based on opinion. Ideally, guidelines should be primarily based on research evidence rather than on opinion; however, guidelines typically have some recommendations based primarily on expert opinion, and these should be labeled as such.

Is the Guideline Applicable to My Practice?

Assuming that the guidelines are primarily evidence based (and that the recommendations which are opinion based are clearly indicated), the user still must decide whether to follow the recommendations.

Is the Burden of Illness Too Low to Warrant Implementation?

If a guideline involves screening for disease, is the risk high enough in your patient population to make this recommendation worthwhile? As discussed in Chapter 8, screening low-risk populations produces far more false positive than true positive test results. Similarly, if the recommendation involves preventive measures, implementing them in a low-risk population may produce more harm than good (Sackett et al. 2000). Guidelines developed for use in tertiary care settings, where the severity of illness and degree of comorbidity are high, may not be applicable in primary care settings, where illness severity is lower (Greenhalgh 2001).

Are the Beliefs of My Patients Incompatible With the Guidelines?

If your patients prefer psychotherapy and the recommendation is for medications (or vice versa), the guideline will be difficult to implement.

Are the Costs and Other Barriers to Implementation Too High?

Perhaps the guideline recommends a type of therapy that is unavailable in your geographic area. Is it practical for someone to be trained in its application? Or perhaps the recommendation concerns a method of delivering services (e.g., assertive community treatment) that is not available in your setting. What are the costs and other barriers to implementation?

■ IMPLEMENTING PRACTICE GUIDELINES

The EBM process described in Chapters 2–4 is one in which individual clinicians search for answers to clinical questions, appraise the evidence, and implement the results. As suggested above and in Chapter 4, clinicians can use evidence-based guidelines as one source of evidence on which to base clinical decisions.

Practice guidelines can also be useful in residency education, although concerns about the quality of some guidelines have made this a controversial issue (Berg et al. 1997). Garfield et al. (2002) recently described their approach to teaching the APA practice guidelines in their psychiatry residency program.

The other use of clinical practice guidelines, and the reason for which guidelines are usually developed, is to attempt to improve the delivery of care within an organization, geographic area, or profession. The results of such attempts have been mixed (Bero et al. 1998; Davis and Taylor-Vaisey 1997; Greenhalgh 2001; Grimshaw and Russell 1993; Grol 2001b; Lipman 2000; National Health Service Centre for Reviews and Dissemination [NHS CRD] 1999; Oxman et al. 1995; Worrall et al. 1997). In general, the passive dissemination of guidelines has little impact on clinical practice (Bero et al. 1998; Davis and TaylorVaisey 1997; Oxman et al. 1995). Guidelines are more apt to be adopted if they take account of local circumstances, are disseminated by active educational interventions, and are implemented using patient-specific reminders (Bero et al. 1998; Feder et al. 1999; Greenhalgh 2001; NHS CRD 1999). Multifaceted interventions tend to be more effective, but they are also more expensive (Bero et al. 1998; Davis and Taylor-Vaisey 1997; Greenhalgh 2001; Grol 1997; NHS CRD 1999; Oxman et al. 1995).

■ REFERENCES

Agency for Health Care Policy and Research: Depression in Primary Care, Vol 1: Detection and Diagnosis. Clinical Practice Guideline No 5. Rockville, MD, U.S. Department of Health and Human Services, 1993a

Agency for Health Care Policy and Research: Depression in Primary Care, Vol 2: Treatment of Major Depression. Clinical Practice Guideline No 5. Rockville, MD, U.S. Department of Health and Human Services, 1993b

American Psychiatric Association: Practice Guidelines for the Treatment of Psychiatric Disorders: Compendium 2002. Washington, DC, American Psychiatric Association, 2002

Antman EM, Lau J, Kupelnick B, et al: A comparison of results of meta-analyses of randomized control trials and recommendations of clinical experts: treatments for myocardial infarction. JAMA 268:240–248, 1992

Badenoch D, Heneghan C: Evidence-Based Medicine Toolkit. London, BMJ Books, 2002

Berg AO, Atkins D, Tierney W: Clinical practice guidelines in practice and education. J Gen Intern Med 12 (suppl 2):S25–S33, 1997

116

Bero LA, Grilli R, Grimshaw JM, et al: Closing the gap between research and practice: an overview of systematic reviews of interventions to promote the implementation of research findings. The Cochrane Effective Practice and Organization of Care Review Group. BMJ 317:465–468, 1998

Birkmeyer JD: Primer on geographic variation in health care. Eff Clin Pract 4:232–233, 2001

Black N, Murphy M, Lamping D, et al: Consensus development methods and their use in creating clinical guidelines, in The Advanced Handbook of Methods in Evidence Based Healthcare. Edited by Stevens A, Abrams K, Brazier J, et al. London, Sage, 2001, pp 426–448

Browman GP: Development and aftercare of clinical guidelines: the balance between rigor and pragmatism. JAMA 286:1509–1511, 2001

Choudhry NK, Stelfox HT, Detsky AS: Relationships between authors of clinical practice guidelines and the pharmaceutical industry. JAMA 287:612–617, 2002

Cook DJ, Greengold NL, Ellrodt AG, et al: The relation between systematic reviews and practice guidelines, in Systematic Reviews: Synthesis of Best Evidence for Health Care Decisions. Edited by Mulrow C, Cook D. Philadelphia, PA, American College of Physicians, 1998, pp 55–65

Davis DA, Taylor-Vaisey A: Translating guidelines into practice: a systematic review of theoretic concepts, practical experience and research evidence in the adoption of clinical practice guidelines. CMAJ 157:408–416, 1997

Drake RE, Goldman HH, Leff HS, et al: Implementing evidence-based practices in routine mental health settings. Psychiatr Serv 52:179–182, 2001

Eccles M, Freemantle N, Mason J: Using systematic reviews in clinical guideline development, in Systematic Reviews in Health Care: Meta-Analysis in Context. Edited by Egger M, Smith GD, Altman DG. London, BMJ Books, 2001, pp 400–409

Expert Consensus Guidelines: Psychiatric treatment guidelines for the most difficult questions facing clinicians [Expert Consensus Guidelines Web site]. April 3, 2002. Available at: http://www.psychguides.com. Accessed September 13, 2002

Feder G, Eccles M, Grol R, et al: Using clinical guidelines. BMJ 318:728–730, 1999

Field MJ, Lohr KN (eds): Clinical Practice Guidelines: Directions for a New Program. Washington, DC, National Academy Press, 1990

Field MJ, Lohr KN (eds): Clinical Practice Guidelines: From Development to Use. Washington, DC, National Academy Press, 1992

Frances A, Kahn D, Carpenter D, et al: A new method of developing expert consensus practice guidelines. American Journal of Managed Care 4:1023–1029, 1998

Garfield D, Atre-Vaidya N, Sierles F: Teaching the APA Practice Guidelines to psychiatry residents: a novel strategy. Acad Psychiatry 26:70–75, 2002

Geddes J, Freemantle N, Harrison P, et al: Atypical antipsychotics in the treatment of schizophrenia: systematic overview and meta-regression analysis. BMJ 321:1371–1376, 2000

Gilbert DA, Altshuler KZ, Rago WV, et al: Texas Medication Algorithm Project: definitions, rationale, and methods to develop medication algorithms. J Clin Psychiatry 59:345–351, 1998

Gray GE: Evidence-based medicine: an introduction for psychiatrists. J Psychiatr Pract 8:5–13, 2002

Greenhalgh T: How to Read a Paper: The Basics of Evidence-Based Medicine, 2nd Edition. London, BMJ Books, 2001

Grimshaw J, Eccles M: Identifying and using evidence-based guidelines in general practice, in Evidence-Based Practice in Primary Care, 2nd Edition. Edited by Silagy C, Haines A. London, BMJ Books, 2001, pp 120–134

Grimshaw JM, Russell IT: Effect of clinical guidelines on medical practice: a systematic review of rigorous evaluations. Lancet 342:1317–1322, 1993

Grol R: Personal paper: beliefs and evidence in changing clinical practice. BMJ 315:418–421, 1997

Grol R: Improving the quality of medical care: building bridges among professional pride, payer profit, and patient satisfaction. JAMA 286:2578–2585, 2001a

Grol R: Successes and failures in the implementation of evidence-based guidelines for clinical practice. Med Care 39 (suppl 2):II-46–II-54, 2001b

Guyatt G, Hayward R, Richardson WS, et al: Moving from evidence to action, in Users' Guides to the Medical Literature: A Manual for Evidence-Based Clinical Practice. Edited by Guyatt G, Rennie D. Chicago, IL, AMA Press, 2002, pp 175–199

Haines A, Jones R: Implementing findings of research. BMJ 308:1488–1492, 1994

Harbour R, Miller J: A new system for grading recommendations in evidence based guidelines. BMJ 323:334–336, 2001

Kahn DA, Docherty JP, Carpenter D, et al: Consensus methods in practice guideline development: a review and description of a new method. Psychopharmacol Bull 33:631–639, 1997

Kapur S, Remington G: Atypical antipsychotics. BMJ 321:1360–1361, 2000

Lehman AF, Steinwachs DM: Patterns of usual care for schizophrenia: initial results from the schizophrenia Patient Outcomes Research Team (PORT) client survey. Schizophr Bull 24:11–20, 1998

Lipman T: Evidence-based practice in general practice and primary care, in Evidence-Based Practice: A Critical Appraisal. Edited by Trinder L, Reynolds S. Oxford, Blackwell Scientific, 2000, pp 35–65

McColl A, Smith H, White P, et al: General practitioners' perception of the route to evidence based medicine: a questionnaire survey. BMJ 316:361–365, 1998

Milner KK, Valenstein M: A comparison of guidelines for the treatment of schizophrenia. Psychiatr Serv 53:888–890, 2002

Mulrow CD: Systematic reviews: rationale for systematic reviews. BMJ 309:597–599, 1994

National Health Service Centre for Reviews and Dissemination: Getting evidence into practice. Eff Health Care 5(1):1–16, 1999

Oxman AD, Thomson MA, Davis DA, et al: No magic bullet: a systematic review of 102 trials of interventions to improve professional practice. CMAJ 153:1423–1431, 1995

Pinsky LE, Deyo RA: Clinical guidelines: a strategy for translating evidence into practice, in Evidence-Based Clinical Practice: Concepts and Approaches. Edited by Geyman JP, Deyo RA, Ramsey SD. Boston, MA, Butterworth-Heinemann, 2000, pp 119–123

Sackett DL, Haynes RB, Guyatt GH, et al: Clinical Epidemiology: A Basic Science for Clinical Medicine, 2nd Edition. Boston, MA, Little, Brown, 1991

Sackett DL, Strauss SE, Richardson WS, et al: Evidence-Based Medicine: How to Practice and Teach EBM, 2nd Edition. New York, Churchill Livingstone, 2000

Shekelle PG, Woolf SH, Eccles M, et al: Developing clinical guidelines. West J Med 170:348–351, 1999a

Shekelle PG, Woolf SH, Eccles M, et al: Developing guidelines. BMJ 318:593–596, 1999b

Shekelle PG, Ortiz E, Rhodes S, et al: Validity of the Agency for Healthcare Research and Quality clinical practice guidelines: how quickly do guidelines become outdated? JAMA 286:1461–1467, 2001

Snowball R: Critical appraisal of clinical guidelines, in Evidence-Based Practice: A Primer for Health Care Professionals. Edited by Dawes M, Davies P, Gray A, et al. Edinburgh, Churchill Livingstone, 1999, pp 127–131

Texas Implementation of Medication Algorithms Web site. January 28, 2003. Available at: http://www.mhmr.state.tx/centraloffice/medical-director/TIMA.html. Accessed June 28, 2003

Texas Medication Algorithm Project: TMAP—a collaborative effort [Texas Medication Algorithm Project Web site]. April 3, 2002. Available at: http://www.mhmr.state.tx.us/centraloffice/medicaldirector/TMAPover .html. Accessed September 13, 2002

Woolf SH, Grol R, Hutchinson A, et al: Potential benefits, limitations, and harms of clinical guidelines. BMJ 318:527–530, 1999a

Woolf SH, Grol R, Hutchinson A, et al: Clinical guidelines: international overview [eBMJ Web site]. February 20, 1999b. Available at: http://bmj.com/cgi/content/full/318/7182/527/DC1/1. Accessed September 24, 2002

Worrall G, Chaulk P, Freake D: The effects of clinical practice guidelines on patient outcomes in primary care: a systematic review. CMAJ 156: 1705–1712, 1997

Young JM, Ward JE: Evidence-based medicine in general practice: beliefs and barriers among Australian GPs. J Eval Clin Pract 7:201–210, 2001

8

DIAGNOSTIC TESTS

Questions about diagnostic tests are most commonly related to the accuracy of the test, which is the focus of this chapter. For information on topics such as the clinical and economic impact of screening, clinical decision rules, and the differential diagnosis process, readers are referred to recent monographs (Hunink et al. 2001; Knottnerus 2002) and standard textbooks of clinical epidemiology (Fletcher et al. 1996; Sackett et al. 1991).

■ EVALUATING DIAGNOSTIC TESTS

The accuracy of a diagnostic test is generally assessed in a cross-sectional study, in which patients are evaluated with both the "gold standard" diagnostic procedure and the diagnostic test under evaluation (Knottnerus and Muris 2002; Knottnerus et al. 2002; Newman et al. 2001). Several important issues can affect the validity of such evaluations (Fletcher et al. 1996; Knottnerus and Muris 2002; Knottnerus et al. 2002; Newman et al. 2001; Sackett et al. 1991), but the two major issues are the choice of the gold standard and the choice of subjects.

Choice of Gold Standard

The first issue is related to the choice of the gold standard. In some branches of medicine, the gold standard might be a pathological diagnosis based on a biopsy or an autopsy; in psychiatry, we rely on the DSM-IV-TR criteria (American Psychiatric Association [APA] 2000a).

Although the DSM-IV-TR diagnostic criteria are often used as the gold standard for evaluating diagnostic tests, they have limitations. First, there are unresolved issues concerning the validity of the criteria themselves (Goldstein and Simpson 2002; Kendell 1989; Kendler 1990).

The second issue relates to the method of eliciting symptoms from patients and of using this information to arrive at a diagnosis. In unstructured clinical interviews, clinicians may ignore or not inquire about certain symptoms and may choose not to follow the DSM criteria in arriving at a diagnosis (Robins 2002). As a result, unstructured interviews may not be reliable. For this reason, a variety of diagnostic instruments have been developed to standardize the process of psychiatric diagnosis, including structured clinical interviews (e.g., the Structured Clinical Interview for DSM-IV [SCID]) and structured interviews that may be administered by either a lay interviewer or a computer (e.g., the Composite International Diagnostic interview [CIDI] and the Diagnostic Interview Schedule [DIS]) (Skodol and Bender 2000). Although these standardized instruments increase the reliability of the diagnoses made, issues of validity remain (Murphy 2002; Narrow et al. 2002; Regier et al. 1998; Robins 2002).

For the assessment of particular symptoms or specific measures of cognitive function (e.g., memory, intelligence, etc.), well-established instruments are generally used as the gold standard. Descriptions of many of these are included in the *Handbook of Psychiatric Measures* (APA 2000b)

Choice of Subjects

The other major issue relates to the choice of subjects. We administer diagnostic tests because we have uncertainty about a diagnosis. A cross-sectional study that includes a spectrum of patients who are similar to those to whom the test is expected to be administered in clinical practice is the most appropriate design. All too often, a test is evaluated in a population composed of a mix of very ill patients and a healthy control group. In such a population, the test performs much better in distinguishing the ill from the healthy than in actual practice. This is referred to as *spectrum bias* (Knottnerus et al. 2002; Newman et al. 2001).

■ MEASURES OF TEST PERFORMANCE: DICHOTOMOUS RESULTS

A variety of terms are used to describe the performance of a diagnostic test (Habbema et al. 2002). As an aid in discussing these terms, Table 8–1 displays the results of a hypothetical comparison of a new diagnostic test with an appropriate gold standard. In this section, we consider test results to be dichotomous (i.e., either positive or negative).

True Positive, True Negative, False Positive, and False Negative

If both the diagnostic test being evaluated and the gold standard yield positive results, the result of the diagnostic test is considered true positive (Table 8–1, cell A). Likewise, if both yield negative results, the result of the diagnostic test is considered true negative (Table 8–1, cell D). If the diagnostic test under evaluation gives a positive result, but the gold standard gives a negative result, the result of the diagnostic test is considered false positive (Table 8–1, cell B). Similarly, if the diagnostic test result is negative, but the gold standard result is positive, the result of the diagnostic test is considered false negative (Table 8–1, cell C).

Sensitivity and Specificity

Sensitivity refers to the proportion of patients with the disease (as assessed by the gold standard) who are detected by the diagnostic test. In Table 8–1, this is calculated as A/(A+C). A highly sensitive test is one that detects most cases of disease.

    Specificity refers to the proportion of patients without the disease (as assessed by the gold standard) who are identified by the

TABLE 8–1. Possible results of a diagnostic test

	Disease present	Disease absent	Totals
Test results positive	A True positive	B False positive	A+B
Test results negative	C False negative	D True negative	C+D
Totals	A+C	B+D	

Sensitivity=A/(A+C)
Specificity=D/(B+D).
Positive predictive value=A/(A+B)
Negative predictive value=D/(C+D)
Likelihood ratio of positive test=[A/(A+C)]/[B/(B+D)]
Likelihood ratio of negative test=[C/(A+C)]/[D/(B+D)]
Error rate=(B+C)/(A+B+C+D)
Accuracy=(A+D)/(A+B+C+D)

diagnostic test as *not* having the disease. In Table 8–1, this is calculated as D/(B+D). A highly specific test is one that does not misidentify healthy individuals as having disease.

Although it may seem counterintuitive, highly sensitive diagnostic tests are most useful for ruling *out* diseases. This is because such tests seldom miss cases of disease. Sackett et al. (2000) have proposed the mnemonic SnNout (**Sen**sitive test, **N**egative result, rules **out** disease) as a teaching aid. Similarly, highly specific tests are most useful for ruling *in* diseases, because they seldom misidentify healthy individuals. The mnemonic for such tests is SpPin (**Sp**ecific test, **P**ositive test, rules **in** disease).

Confidence intervals (CIs) for specificity and sensitivity can be calculated using the tables given by Habbema et al. (2002).

Positive and Negative Predictive Values

The positive predictive value (PPV) is the proportion of positive test results that is true positives. Using Table 8–1, PPV is calculated as A/(A+B). The negative predictive value (NPV) is the proportion of negative test results that is true negatives. Using Table 8–1, NPV is calculated as D/(C+D).

PPV and NPV can also be looked at in terms of posttest probabilities of disease (Fletcher et al. 1996; Habbema et al. 2002). PPV represents the probability that an individual with a positive test result has the disease, whereas NPV represents the probability that an individual with a negative test result does not have the disease.

PPV and NPV are dependent on the prevalence of disease in the population being tested, which is also referred to as the *pretest probability of disease* (Fletcher et al. 1996). Mathematically, the relationship is as follows:

$$PPV = \frac{\text{sensitivity} \times \text{prevalence}}{(\text{sensitivity} \times \text{prevalence}) + [(1 - \text{specificity})(1 - \text{prevalence})]}$$

Because of this dependence on disease prevalence, screening for diseases in low-prevalence populations yields few true-positive test results, regardless of the sensitivity and specificity of the test (Fletcher et al. 1996). Baldessarini et al. (1983) have provided an excellent discussion of the effects of disease prevalence on PPV in psychiatric practice, using as their example the dexamethasone suppression test as a diagnostic test for depression.

Likelihood Ratios

Although PPV and NPV allow the clinician to estimate the probability of disease in a patient with a particular test result, they are both dependent on the prevalence of disease in the study population. Likelihood ratios (LRs), in contrast, are independent of disease prevalence.

The likelihood ratio of a positive test (LR+) is the ratio of the likelihood (probability) of a positive test result in the population with disease divided by the likelihood of a positive test result in the population without disease. This can be calculated as follows, using the data in Table 8–1:

$$LR+ = \frac{A/(A+C)}{B/B+D} = \frac{\text{sensitivity}}{1 - \text{specificity}}$$

The likelihood ratio of a negative test result (LR–) is similarly the ratio of the likelihood of a negative test result in the population with disease divided by the likelihood of a negative test result in the population without disease. Once again, using the data in Table 8–1:

$$LR- = \frac{C/(A+C)}{D/(B+D)} = \frac{1 - \text{sensitivity}}{\text{specificity}}$$

Formulas for calculating CIs for LRs are given by Habbema et al. (2002).

One of the most useful features of LRs is that they can be used to estimate the probability that a given patient has an illness, given a particular test result. The following formula can be used for this estimate:

$$\text{posttest odds } = \text{ pretest odds} \times \text{LR}$$

As mentioned in Chapter 5, the odds of an event occurring is the ratio of the probability of an event occurring (P) divided by the probability of the event not occurring ($1-P$), or the odds $= P/(1-P)$.

The pretest probability of disease in a patient can be estimated from the prevalence of a disease in your own or similar patient populations, as derived from papers evaluating diagnostic tests, epidemiologic studies, or hospital statistics (Mant 1999; Sackett et al. 2000). For some medical conditions, clinical prediction rules may be used to better refine the estimated pretest probability (McGinn 2002). Sometimes published data are not available and a subjective estimate of pretest probability must be made, although this is subject to numerous biases (Elstein and Schwartz 2002; Hunink et al. 2001). When there is uncertainty about the pretest probability, it is best to estimate an upper and lower limit and to do the calculations with both values to see if it will change your management of the patient.

Once you have a pretest probability of disease, it is converted to the pretest odds, using the formula above. The pretest odds are then multiplied by the appropriate likelihood ratio (LR+ if the test is positive or LR– if the test is negative). The resulting posttest odds can then be converted to a posttest probability, using the following formula:

$$P = \frac{\text{odds}}{1+\text{odds}}$$

For those wishing to go directly from pretest probability to posttest probability, without having to go back and forth between probabilities and odds, nomograms and computer programs are available (Fagan 1975; Glasziou 2001).

Using diagnostic tests in this way to quantify the risk of disease in a patient and to then use these probabilities in clinical decision making has become an important field of study, but it is outside of the scope this chapter. For further details, readers are referred to the recent text of Hunink et al. (2001) and the accounts of Sackett et al. (1991, 2000).

Error Rate and Accuracy

The error rate of a diagnostic test is the percentage of test results that is either false positives or false negatives (Habbema et al. 2002). Using the data in Table 8–1, error rate can be calculated as follows:

$$\frac{B+C}{A+B+C+D}$$

The term *accuracy* is sometimes used to describe the percentage of test results that is either true positives or true negatives (Fletcher et al. 1996; Greenhalgh 2001). Using the data in Table 8–1, it is calculated as follows:

$$\frac{A+D}{A+B+C+D}$$

Accuracy can also be calculated as 1−error rate.

Diagnostic Odds Ratio

The diagnostic odds ratio (DOR) is sometimes used as a measure of overall test performance (Habbema et al. 2002). Using the data in Table 8–1, it is calculated as follows:

$$\frac{A \times D}{B \times C}$$

The DOR is sometimes used in systematic reviews and in meta-analyses because of its mathematical properties; however, it is not a statistic that is easy to interpret clinically (Deeks 2001).

Example of Calculations

Table 8–2 provides data from a study by Watkins et al. (2001) that evaluates the accuracy of a single question ("Do you feel sad or depressed?") in screening for depression in stroke patients. In the study, answers to the question ("yes" or "no") were compared with the results of the Montgomery-Åsberg Rating Depression Rating Scale (MADRS), with a MADRS score >6 indicating depression. As can be seen from Table 8–2, the single question had a sensitivity of 86% and a specificity of 78%.

We can use LRs to see the impact of a positive or negative response to the question on the probability of a patient being depressed. Depression typically occurs in 25%–40% of patients with stroke and other neurologic conditions (APA 2000a). Thus, the pretest odds for such a patient are between $25/75=0.33$ and $40/60=0.67$. If the patient answers "yes" to the question, the posttest odds are between $0.33 \times 3.87=1.29$ and $0.67 \times 3.87=2.58$, corresponding to posttest probabilities of 56%–72%. If the patient answers "no," the posttest odds are between $0.33 \times 0.18=0.06$ and $0.67 \times 0.18=0.12$, corresponding to posttest probabilities of 6%–11%.

■ MEASURES OF TEST PERFORMANCE: ORDINAL OR CONTINUOUS RESULTS

Although we often think of diagnostic test results as positive or negative, rating scales and many laboratory tests have more than just two values. Rating scales, for example, can have outcomes that are ordered categories (e.g., none, minimal, mild, moderate, or severe) or that yield a numerical score. Although a cutoff value is often chosen to convert such an outcome to a dichotomous measure, information is lost in the process.

Choosing a Cutoff Score

When a test result can take more than two values as described above, a decision must be made about a cutoff score if the results

TABLE 8–2. Accuracy of a single question ("Do you often feel sad or depressed?") in screening for depression in stroke patients

Answer to question	Depressed (MADRS>6)	Not depressed (MADRS ≤6)	Totals
Yes	37	8	45
No	6	28	34
Totals	43	36	79

Sensitivity=37/43=86%
Specificity=28/36=78%
Positive predictive value=37/45=82%
Negative predictive value=28/34=82%
Likelihood ratio of positive test=0.86/0.22=3.9
Likelihood ratio of negative test=0.14/0.78=0.18
Error rate=14/79=18%
Accuracy=65/79=82%

Note. MADRS=Montgomery-Åsberg Depression Rating Scale.
Source. Data from Watkins et al. 2001.

TABLE 8–3.	Sensitivity and specificity of the CAGE questionnaire in screening for alcohol abuse in general medical patients	

CAGE score cutoff	Sensitivity (%)	Specificity (%)
0 vs. 1+	89	81
<2 vs. 2+	74	91
<3 vs. 3+	44	98
<4 vs. 4+	25	100

Source. Data from Buchsbaum et al. 1991.

are to be viewed as either positive or negative. The choice of the cutoff value involves a trade-off between sensitivity and specificity (Fletcher et al. 1996).

Table 8–3 shows the results of a study of the CAGE questionnaire as a screening tool for diagnosing alcohol abuse in general medical patients (Buchsbaum et al. 1991). (CAGE is an acronym for certain key symptoms of alcohol abuse.) As can be seen, as the cutoff score is increased, the specificity increases, but the sensitivity decreases. At the usual cutoff score of 2 (Rounsaville and Poling 2000), the sensitivity is 74% and the specificity is 91%.

Receiver Operator Characteristic Curves

The data in Table 8–3 can also be displayed graphically, in the form of a receiver operator characteristic (ROC) curve (Figure 8–1). An ROC curve plots the sensitivity against (1−specificity) for each cutoff value (Fletcher et al. 1996; Sackett et al. 1991, 2000). The ROC curve can be used to identify a cutoff value, where a point near the upper left corner is the appropriate cutoff. ROC curves can also be used to compare two diagnostic tests; the better test is the one with its ROC curve closer to the upper left corner (Fletcher et al. 1996).

Likelihood Ratios

Intuitively, it would seem that converting numerical or ordered test results into just two categories would result in a loss of in-

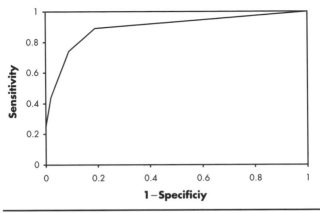

FIGURE 8–1. **Receiver operator characteristic curve for CAGE questionnaire.**

Source. Data from Buchsbaum et al. (1991).

formation. It would seem that a value greatly over the cutoff would be more indicative of disease than a value that is barely more than the cutoff. LRs allow these differences to be taken into account.

If a test result takes multiple values, LRs can be calculated for multiple scores, not just LR+ and LR–. This is illustrated in Table 8–4, using the same CAGE data found in Table 8–3 (Buchsbaum et al. 1991). It can be seen that as the CAGE score increases from 0 to 4, LRs increase from 0.14 to 100. Assuming a prevalence (pretest probability) of alcohol dependence of 5% (APA 2000a), a CAGE score of 0 decreases the posttest probability to 1%. Using the same figures, a CAGE score of 2 increases the posttest probability to 19% and a CAGE score of 5 increases the posttest probability to 84%. Clearly, this provides more information than simply treating the results as *positive* (2+) or *negative* (0–1).

TABLE 8–4.   Likelihood ratios for specific CAGE scores in
screening for alcohol abuse in general
medical patients

CAGE score	Likelihood ratio
0	0.14
1	1.5
2	4.5
3	13
4	100

Source.   Data from Buchsbaum et al. 1991.

■ SYSTEMATIC REVIEWS AND META-ANALYSES OF DIAGNOSTIC TESTS

As with the evaluation of therapies, systematic reviews that are related to diagnostic tests may be conducted. However, there are several approaches to meta-analysis (Deeks 2001; Glasziou et al. 2001). One approach is to use one forest plot for sensitivities and their CIs and another forest plot for specificities and their CIs (see Chapter 6). Another approach is to plot the sensitivity against (1 – specificity) on an ROC plot, with each study representing one point on the plot. Methods deriving pooled estimates of sensitivity, specificity, and LRs are also available. Finally, DORs can be pooled and this can be used to derive a summary ROC curve. Although such methods can demonstrate that a test is useful, if there is heterogeneity in results the summary statistics may not give a valid estimate of the probability associated with a specific test outcome (Deeks 2001).

■ CRITICAL APPRAISAL GUIDE FOR STUDIES OF DIAGNOSTIC TEST ACCURACY

Having discussed how diagnostic tests are evaluated and measures of their accuracy, we now turn to the critical appraisal of reports of

TABLE 8–5.	Critical appraisal guide for studies of diagnostic accuracy

Is the study valid?

Is it a cross-sectional study?

Was the test evaluated in an appropriate spectrum of patients?

Was there an independent blind comparison with a "gold standard"?

Were both tests administered, regardless of outcome?

Are the results important?

What is the sensitivity?

What is the specificity?

What is the positive predictive value?

What is the negative predictive value?

What is the likelihood ratio for a positive test result?

What is the likelihood ratio for a negative test result?

Can I apply the results to my patient?

Is the test available or feasible in my setting?

Do I have enough information to apply the test and to interpret the results?

Given reasonable pretest estimates of disease probability in my patient, what are the posttest probabilities if the test is positive? If it is negative?

Will these probabilities change my management of the patient?

Source.   Based on Gilbert et al. 2001; Glasziou et al. 2001; Sackett et al. 2000.

such evaluations. A guide for critically appraising studies of diagnostic test accuracy is given in Table 8–5.

Is the Study Valid?

As discussed earlier in this chapter, the appropriate study design to assess the accuracy of a diagnostic test is a cross-sectional study in which patients are evaluated with both the gold standard diagnostic procedure and the diagnostic test under evaluation (Knottnerus and Muris 2002; Knottnerus et al. 2002; Newman et al. 2001). Both tests should be administered blindly to avoid observer bias (Fletcher et al. 1996), and the results of one test should not influence the decision to administer the other test. The gold standard itself should be appropriate, and an appropriate spectrum of patients should be chosen to avoid "spectrum bias" (Knottnerus et al. 2002; Newman et al. 2001).

Are the Results Important?

Sensitivity and specificity are the usual measures of diagnostic test accuracy. Which of the two is more important will depend on the purpose of the test. Recall that highly sensitive diagnostic tests are most useful for ruling *out* diseases (SnNout: **Sen**sitive test, **N**egative result, rules **out** disease), whereas highly specific tests are most useful for ruling *in* diseases (SpPin: **Sp**ecific test, **P**ositive test, rules **in** disease) (Sackett et al. 2000).

PPV and NPV will provide estimates of the probabilities of disease in patients with positive or negative test results, respectively, in the study population. However, LR+ and LR– are more useful measures, because they can be generalized to other populations with different disease prevalences (Fletcher et al. 1996; Mant 1999).

Can I Apply the Results to My Patient?

The first question to ask is whether the test is feasible in your setting. Does it require specialized equipment or is it very expensive? Does it require expertise to administer or to interpret the test, and is such expertise available?

The next question is specific to your patient and relates to whether the results of the test will change your patient management. As described in more detail elsewhere (Hunink et al. 2001; Sackett et al. 1991, 2000), physicians make decisions about clinical management, based on their (often unstated) assessments of the probability of disease in a given patient. If that probability is high, physicians treat the patient; if that probability is intermediate, physicians order more diagnostic tests; and if it is low, physicians do neither. The probability at or above which tests are ordered is termed the *test threshold*, and the probability at or above which treatment is begun is termed the *treatment threshold* (Hunink et al. 2001; Sackett et al. 2000).

If your patient's pretest probability is already above the treatment threshold, there is no point in ordering the diagnostic test. For example, if your diagnostic interview shows that your patient met the DSM-IV-TR criteria for major depression, there is no need to also use a rating scale developed to screen for depression. You have already established the diagnosis with enough certainty to begin treatment.

Conversely, if the posttest probability remains low even if the test result is positive, the test should probably not be performed because it is likely that any positive test result will be a false positive. Ordering the test under these circumstances would be both a waste of money and an unnecessary cause of anxiety for patients with false-positive results (Fletcher et al. 1996).

To do these sorts of calculations, you will need the LR+ and LR− from the article reporting the performance of the test in question and an estimate of your patient's pretest probability of disease. If your patient is similar to patients in the study population, the pretest probability can be derived from the study evaluating the diagnostic test. If not, the pretest probability can be estimated from epidemiologic data or from patient data from your hospital or health maintenance organization (Mant 1999; Sackett et al. 2000). If published data are not available, you may have to make a subjective estimate of the pretest. In this case, it is probably best to estimate an upper and lower limit and to do the calculations with both values.

If the test is valid and feasible and if the results will make a difference in patient management, you should use it and then proceed to the next step in the EBM process (see Chapter 12).

■ REFERENCES

American Psychiatric Association: Diagnostic and Statistical Manual of Mental Disorders, 4th Edition, Text Revision. Washington, DC, American Psychiatric Association, 2000a

American Psychiatric Association: Handbook of Psychiatric Measures. Washington, DC, American Psychiatric Association, 2000b

Baldessarini RJ, Finkelstein S, Arana GW: The predictive power of diagnostic tests and the effect of prevalence of illness. Arch Gen Psychiatry 40:569–573, 1983

Buchsbaum DG, Buchanan RG, Centor RM, et al: Screening for alcohol abuse using CAGE scores and likelihood ratios. Ann Intern Med 115:774–777, 1991

Deeks JJ: Systematic reviews of evaluation of diagnostic and screening tests. BMJ 323:157–162, 2001

Elstein AS, Schwartz A: Clinical problem solving and diagnostic decision making: a selective review of the cognitive research literature, in The Evidence Base of Clinical Diagnosis. Edited by Knottnerus JA. London, BMJ Books, 2002, pp 179–195

Fagan TJ: Nomogram for Bayes' theorem. N Engl J Med 293:257, 1975

Fletcher RH, Fletcher SW, Wagner EH: Clinical Epidemiology: The Essentials, 3rd Edition. Baltimore, MD, Williams & Wilkins, 1996

Gilbert R, Logan S, Moyer VA, et al: Assessing diagnostic and screening tests, II: how to use the research literature on diagnosis. West J Med 175:37–41, 2001

Glasziou P: Which methods for bedside Bayes? ACP J Club 135:A11–A12, 2001

Glasziou P, Irwig L, Bain C, et al; Systematic Reviews in Health Care: A Practical Guide. Cambridge, UK, Cambridge University Press, 2001

Goldstein JM, Simpson JC: Validity: definitions and applications to psychiatric research, in Textbook of Psychiatric Epidemiology, 2nd Edition. Edited by Tsuang MT, Tohen M. New York, Wiley-Liss, 2002, pp 149–163

Greenhalgh T: How to Read a Paper: The Basics of Evidence Based Medicine, 2nd Edition. London, BMJ Books, 2001

Habbema JDF, Eijkemans R, Krijnen P, et al: Analysis of data on the accuracy of diagnostic tests, in The Evidence Base of Clinical Diagnosis. Edited by Knottnerus JA. London, BMJ Books, 2002, pp 117–143

Hunink M, Glasziou P, Siegel J, et al: Decision Making in Health and Medicine: Integrating Evidence and Values. New York, Cambridge University Press, 2001

Kendell RE: Clinical validity. Psychol Med 19:45–55, 1989

Kendler KS: Toward a scientific psychiatric nosology: strengths and limitations. Arch Gen Psychiatry 47:969–973, 1990

Knottnerus JA (ed): The Evidence Base of Clinical Diagnosis. London, BMJ Books, 2002

Knottnerus JA, Muris JWM: Assessment of the accuracy of diagnostic tests: the cross-sectional study, in The Evidence Base of Clinical Diagnosis. Edited by Knottnerus JA. London, BMJ Books, 2002, pp 39–60

Knottnerus JA, van Weel C, Muris JWM: Evaluation of diagnostic procedures. BMJ 324:477–480, 2002

Mant J: Is this test effective? In Evidence-Based Practice: A Primer for Health Professionals. Edited by Dawes M, Davies P, Gray A, et al. New York, Churchill Livingstone, 1999, pp 133–157

McGinn T: Practice corner: using clinical prediction rules. ACP J Club 137:A10–A11, 2002

Murphy JM: Symptom scales and diagnostic schedules in adult psychiatry, in Textbook of Psychiatric Epidemiology, 2nd Edition. Edited by Tsuang MT, Tohen M. New York, Wiley-Liss, 2002, pp 273–332

Narrow WE, Rae DS, Robins LN, et al: Revised prevalence estimates of mental disorders in the United States: using a clinical significance criterion to reconcile 2 surveys' estimates. Arch Gen Psychiatry 59:115–123, 2002

Newman TB, Browner WS, Cummings SR: Designing studies of medical tests, in Designing Clinical Research, 2nd Edition. Edited by Hulley SB, Cummings SR, Browner WS, et al. Philadelphia, PA, Lippincott Williams and Wilkins, 2001, pp 175–191

Regier DA, Kaelber CT, Rae DS, et al: Limitations of diagnostic criteria and assessment instruments for mental disorders: implications for research and policy. Arch Gen Psychiatry 55:109–115, 1998

Robins LN: Birth and development of psychiatric interviews, in Textbook of Psychiatric Epidemiology, 2nd Edition. Edited by Tsuang MT, Tohen M. New York, Wiley-Liss, 2002, pp 257–271

Rounsaville BJ, Poling J: Substance use disorders measures, in Handbook of Psychiatric Measures. Washington, DC, American Psychiatric Association, 2000, pp 457–484

Sackett DL, Haynes RB, Guyatt GH, et al: Clinical Epidemiology: A Basic Science for Clinical Medicine, 2nd Edition. Boston, MA, Little, Brown, 1991

Sackett DL, Strauss SE, Richardson WS, et al: Evidence-Based Medicine: How to Practice and Teach EBM, 2nd Edition. New York, Churchill Livingstone, 2000

Skodol AE, Bender DS: Diagnostic interviews for adults, in Handbook of Psychiatric Measures. Washington, DC, American Psychiatric Association, 2000, pp 45–70

Watkins C, Daniels L, Jack C, et al: Accuracy of a single question in screening for depression in a cohort of patients after stroke: comparative study. BMJ 323:1159, 2001

9

SURVEYS OF DISEASE FREQUENCY

Questions about disease frequency take various forms. A patient's family member or member of the public may wonder about the risk of developing a disease. An administrator may wonder about the number of patients who will need treatment. A clinician attempting to evaluate a patient's risk of disease, based on the results of a diagnostic test, will need information on the patient's pretest probability of disease (see Chapter 8).

All of these questions require quantitative information about the frequency of a particular illness in a defined population of interest, which is the subject of descriptive epidemiology. This chapter reviews the various measures of disease frequency and the methods of descriptive epidemiology, as background information for the critical appraisal of studies of disease frequency. For additional information, readers are referred to standard epidemiology texts (Fletcher et al. 1996; Gordis 2000; Hennekens et al. 1987; Lilienfeld and Stolley 1994) and reviews of psychiatric epidemiology (Regier and Burke 2000; Tsuang and Tohen 2002).

■ MEASURES OF DISEASE FREQUENCY

A number of terms, such as *incidence*, *prevalence*, and *lifetime prevalence*, are used—and often misused—to refer to the frequency of disease in a population.

Incidence

The *incidence* of disease is the number of new cases of disease in a defined population in a given period of time. It is measured by starting with a population (cohort) that is initially free of the disease in question and by then counting the cases that develop in a defined period of time. The incidence rate has "cases" as its numerator and "person-years at risk " as its denominator. The incidence rate is the measure of frequency of most interest to epidemiologists seeking to understand the cause of a disease, because it measures the actual risk of developing the disease.

Point Prevalence

When epidemiologists use the term *prevalence*, they are usually referring to the *point prevalence* (i.e., the number of cases of disease in a defined population at a given point in time). It is measured in a cross-sectional survey in which individuals are identified as either having or not having a disease at the time of the survey.

Point prevalence is of interest to health care planners, because it measures the burden of illness in a population. It is also of interest to clinicians, because it is a measure of a patient's pretest probability of disease (see Chapter 8).

Point prevalence is less helpful in understanding the causes of disease, because it reflects both the incidence (risk) of disease and the duration of the illness. In a *steady state* situation in which the incidence rate and average duration of illness are constant, the following relationship between incidence and point prevalence exists:

point prevalence = incidence rate × average duration of illness

This relationship allows for the calculation of the third variable in the equation, if the other two variables are known.

Period Prevalence

Period prevalence is a measure of the proportion of individuals in a defined population who have an illness in a specified period of time. It is a hybrid measure that reflects both the proportion of patients who have the illness at the start of the time interval (prevalence), as well as the number of new cases that develop during the time period (incidence × time).

Although period prevalence is seldom used outside psychiatry (Hennekens et al. 1987), it is widely used in surveys of the frequency of psychiatric illnesses (Fleming and Hsieh 2002; Regier and Burke 2000). In the National Comorbidity Survey, for example, results were reported as 12-month prevalences, which indicates that an individual had the disorder in question at some time during the 12 months prior to the interview date (Kessler and Walters 2002).

The popularity of period prevalence in psychiatric epidemiology relates to the fact that many psychiatric illnesses have a recurring or episodic course; therefore, the period prevalence is believed to be a better reflection of disease burden in the population than is the proportion of patients who are symptomatic at a given point in time.

Lifetime Prevalence

Lifetime prevalence is a specific type of period prevalence used in psychiatric epidemiology. As used in the National Comorbidity Survey and in similar studies, *lifetime prevalence* is the proportion of the patients in population studies who have experienced an illness up to the point in their life that they are surveyed.

Defined in this way, lifetime prevalence has several limitations (Fleming and Hsieh 2002; Regier and Burke 2000). First, it is dependent on memory (recall bias). Second, it is highly dependent on the age structure of the population, with young people less likely to develop the disease than older people. Third, if the disease is associated with excess mortality from suicide or other causes, lifetime prevalence may decline with age.

Morbidity Risk

An alternative measure of lifetime risk, sometimes referred to as *lifetime expectancy*, is morbidity risk or morbid risk (Faraone et al. 2002; Slater and Cowie 1971). This measure corrects the denominator to reflect the fact that younger individuals have had less chance to develop the illness than older individuals and is a better estimate of the risk of developing the illness at some point during a normal lifespan.

Age- and Sex-Specific and Adjusted Rates

The incidence and prevalence of many psychiatric disorders vary with age and sex. The incidence of major depression, for example, is greater in women than in men (Horwath et al. 2002), and the incidence and prevalence of dementia increase with age, beginning at about age 65 years (Hybels and Blazer 2002). In determining the pretest probability of disease for an individual, using age- and sex-specific prevalences will be more accurate than using the prevalence figures for the population as a whole.

When comparing rates between geographic areas or over time, it is important to take demographic differences into account. For example, differences in the incidence of depression in two populations could reflect actual differences in risk for disease or they could simply reflect differences in age or sex distribution. To eliminate demographic differences as the explanation, rates can be standardized. In essence, this involves calculating a weighted average of the age- and sex-specific rates, using identical weights for both populations. Methods of standardization and details of the calculations can be found in standard epidemiology and biostatistics texts (Gordis 2000; Hennekens et al. 1987; Pagano and Gauvreau 2000).

Using Registries and Existing Records

There are several potential sources of existing or routinely collected information about the frequency of disease in a population. These resources include disease registries, reporting systems, and insurance or health plan statistics (Gordis 2000; Lilienfeld and Stolley 1994).

For some diseases (e.g., cancer and some infectious diseases), established disease reporting systems and case registries can provide considerable information about incidence or prevalence. In psychiatry, largely because of privacy concerns, such registers or reporting systems are largely nonexistent. Notable exceptions to this include case registers of psychiatric cases in Rochester, NY; in Denmark; and in Mannheim, Germany (Regier and Burke 2000). Information from such registers is largely limited to schizophrenia and to other serious mental illnesses that require hospitalization.

Records maintained by a health maintenance organization or a health plan can be used to provide useful information about the treated prevalence of mental illness in the health plan's members. Unfortunately, much illness goes untreated, so such records underestimate the actual frequency of mental illness in the health plan's members. As a result, surveys are required to better estimate the actual frequency of disease in a population.

■ SURVEYS OF DISEASE FREQUENCY

Two aspects of the design of surveys that are used to determine the incidence or prevalence of a disease in a population are of particular importance: who to survey and how to assess the presence of absence of disease.

Populations and Samples

The first decision involves deciding on the population of interest (Hulley et al. 2001). Although we often are interested in the frequency of disease in the general population, the prevalence of many psychiatric disorders is greater in specific settings (e.g., primary care settings or jails) and can vary with ethnicity (Burke 2002). Thus, there is a rationale for conducting surveys among subpopulations and in specific settings, as well as in the general population.

After deciding on the population of interest, the next step is to assemble a sample of individuals to actually study. A variety of techniques can be used for this purpose (Hulley et al. 2001). If the population is such that all members can be enumerated (e.g., members of a health plan), a simple random sample can be used. For community surveys, cluster sampling is often used. In cluster sampling, the investigators first randomly select census tracts or similar geographic areas, followed by a sample of addresses within the geographic area. Details of the various sampling methods, including methods of determining the sample size required for a certain precision in the estimate of the prevalence rate, can be found in standard texts on survey methods (Kalton 1983; Kelsey et al. 1996).

Assessment Instrument

The second decision relates to the method used to decide whether an individual has the disease of interest or not. Although we use the DSM-IV-TR diagnostic criteria (American Psychiatric Association [APA] 2000a), we must also have a method of eliciting symptoms and for applying these criteria during a survey. The chosen method must be feasible, reliable, and valid (Regier and Burke 2000).

Reliability refers to the ability of an assessment instrument to yield a consistent result. In unstructured clinical interviews, clinicians may ignore or not inquire about certain symptoms and may choose not to follow DSM criteria in arriving at a diagnosis (Robins 2002). As a result, unstructured interviews may not be reliable. As noted in Chapter 8, a variety of diagnostic instruments have been developed to standardize and improve the reliability of the psychiatric diagnosis process, including structured interviews, administered either by a clinician (e.g., the Structured Clinical Interview for DSM-IV [SCID]) or by a lay interviewer (e.g., the Composite International Diagnostic Interview [CIDI] and the Diagnostic Interview Schedule [DIS]) (Skodol and Bender 2000).

The other issue is *validity* (i.e., whether the instrument measures its intended parameters). Although the standardized instruments mentioned above have improved the reliability of the diagnoses made in surveys, issues of validity remain (Murphy

2002; Regier et al. 1998; Robins 2002). In particular, community surveys identify individuals who have less severe symptoms than those seen among individuals in treatment settings, and it is unclear if these represent milder cases of the same disorders or simply non-pathological transient responses to stressors (Narrow et al. 2002; Regier et al. 1998).

For the assessment of particular symptoms or specific measures of cognitive function (e.g., memory, intelligence, etc.), a variety of well-established instruments that are considered both reliable and valid are available. Descriptions of many of these are included in the *Handbook of Psychiatric Measures* (APA 2000b).

■ CRITICAL APPRAISAL OF A SURVEY OF DISEASE FREQUENCY

Having discussed the various measures of disease frequency and how they are determined, we now turn to the critical appraisal of reports of disease frequency. A guide for critically appraising these studies is given in Table 9–1.

Is the Study Valid?

The first questions relate to the study design. For estimating prevalence, a cross-sectional survey, in which individuals are identified as either having or not having a disease either at the time of the survey or during some defined time period, is the appropriate design. Incidence rates are measured in cohort studies, in which a group of individuals who are initially free of the disease in question is followed over time, and cases of disease that develop in the cohort during the follow-up period are counted.

Regardless of study design, the individuals surveyed should be members of a defined population that is sampled in such a way as to give an unbiased estimate or incidence or prevalence rate. A convenience sample or the use of volunteers recruited from an advertisement cannot be considered representative of a defined population; it will give a biased estimate of disease frequency, which is

TABLE 9–1.	Critical appraisal guide for surveys of disease frequency

Is the study valid?

Is the study design appropriate (cross-sectional survey for measuring prevalence or cohort study for measuring incidence)?

Was an appropriate sampling method used?

Was the response rate sufficiently high?

Was a standardized method used to determine the presence of disease?

Is the assessment instrument reliable and valid?

Are the results important?

What is the incidence or prevalence?

Are there important differences by age, sex, ethnicity, etc.?

How precise are the estimates?

Can I apply the results to my patient?

Does my patient come from a population similar to that surveyed?

Are there age- or sex-specific estimates (if appropriate) that apply to my patient?

Source.   Based in part on the criteria of Barker et al. 1998; Fletcher et al. 1996.

referred to as *selection bias* (Daly and Bourke 2000).

Nonresponse bias is an additional concern, because individuals who refuse to participate in the survey may be systematically different from individuals who do participate (Aday 1996; Barker et al. 1998; Daly and Bourke 2000). For example, telephone followup of nonresponders in the National Comorbidity Survey found that they were more apt to have an anxiety disorder than were responders (Kessler and Walters 2002). In general, it is considered desirable to have as high a response rate as possible—generally, at least 75%–80% (Aday 1996; Barker et al. 1998; Kelsey et al. 1996).

It is essential to use standard criteria to decide whether an individual has a disorder or not, because the prevalence will depend on the definition of what constitutes a case (Fletcher et al. 1996). In addition, as described above under "Surveys of Disease Frequency," the assessment instrument must have acceptable reliability and validity (Regier and Burke 2000).

Are the Results Important?

Which results are important will, of course, be related to your initial clinical question. At a minimum, you would expect to see an incidence or prevalence rate for each disorder surveyed, with confidence limits. If your goal is to apply the results to an individual patient, rates specific to age, sex, and other demographic characteristics will be helpful. In contrast, if your interest lies in comparing the rates in two populations, standardized rates will be of more interest.

Can I Apply the Results to My Patient?

The first question to ask is whether the population is similar enough that the results can reasonably be generalized to your patient (Hulley et al. 2001). In addition, if your clinical question relates to a pretest probability of disease in your patient (see Chapter 8), the availability of age- and sex-specific prevalence rates will give you a more accurate estimate than will crude or standardized rates.

■ REFERENCES

Aday LA: Designing and Conducting Health Surveys: A Comprehensive Guide, 2nd Edition. San Francisco, CA, Jossey-Bass, 1996

American Psychiatric Association: Diagnostic and Statistical Manual of Mental Disorders, 4th Edition, Text Revision. Washington, DC, American Psychiatric Association, 2000a

American Psychiatric Association: Handbook of Psychiatric Measures. Washington, DC, American Psychiatric Association, 2000b

Barker DJP, Cooper C, Rose G: Epidemiology in Medical Practice, 5th Edition. New York, Churchill Livingstone, 1998

Burke JD: Mental health services research, in Textbook in Psychiatric Epidemiology, 2nd Edition. Edited by Tsuang MT, Tohen M. New York, Wiley-Liss, 2002, pp 165–179

Daly LE, Bourke GJ: Interpretation and Uses of Medical Statistics, 5th Edition. Oxford, UK, Blackwell Scientific, 2000

Faraone SV, Tsuang D, Tsuang MT: Methods in psychiatric genetics, in Textbook in Psychiatric Epidemiology, 2nd Edition. Edited by Tsuang MT, Tohen M. New York, Wiley-Liss, 2002, pp 65–130

Fleming JA, Hsieh C-C: Introduction to epidemiologic research methods, in Textbook in Psychiatric Epidemiology, 2nd Edition. Edited by Tsuang MT, Tohen M. New York, Wiley-Liss, 2002, pp 3–33

Fletcher RH, Fletcher SW, Wagner EH: Clinical Epidemiology: The Essentials, 3rd Edition. Baltimore, MD, Williams & Wilkins, 1996

Gordis L: Epidemiology, 2nd Edition. Philadelphia, PA, WB Saunders, 2000

Hennekens CH, Buring JE, Mayrent SL: Epidemiology in Medicine. Boston, MA, Little, Brown, 1987

Horwath E, Cohen RS, Weissman MM: Epidemiology of depressive and anxiety disorders, in Textbook in Psychiatric Epidemiology, 2nd Edition. Edited by Tsuang MT, Tohen M. New York, Wiley-Liss, 2002, pp 389–426

Hulley SB, Newman TB, Cummings SR: Choosing the study subjects: specification, sampling, and recruitment, in Designing Clinical Research: An Epidemiologic Approach, 2nd Edition. Edited by Hulley SB, Cummings SR, Browner WS, et al. Philadelphia, PA, Lippincott Williams & Williams, 2001, pp 25–36

Hybels CF, Blazer DG: Epidemiology and geriatric psychiatry, in Textbook in Psychiatric Epidemiology, 2nd Edition. Edited by Tsuang MT, Tohen M. New York, Wiley-Liss, 2002, pp 603–628

Kalton G: Introduction to Survey Sampling. Newbury Park, CA, Sage, 1983

Kelsey JL, Whittemore AS, Evans AS, et al (eds): Methods in Observational Epidemiology, 2nd Edition. New York, Oxford University Press, 1996

Kessler RC, Walters E: The National Comorbidity Survey, in Textbook in Psychiatric Epidemiology, 2nd Edition. Edited by Tsuang MT, Tohen M. New York, Wiley-Liss, 2002, pp 343–362

Lilienfeld DE, Stolley PD: Foundations of Epidemiology, 3rd Edition. New York, Oxford University Press, 1994

Murphy JM: Symptom scales and diagnostic schedules in adult psychiatry, in Textbook of Psychiatric Epidemiology, 2nd Edition. Edited by Tsuang MT, Tohen M. New York, Wiley-Liss, 2002, pp 273–332

Narrow WE, Rae DS, Robins LN, et al: Revised prevalence estimates of mental disorders in the United States: using a clinical significance criterion to reconcile 2 surveys' estimates. Arch Gen Psychiatry 59:115–123, 2002

Pagano M, Gauvreau K: Principles of Biostatistics, 2nd Edition. Pacific Grove, CA, Duxbury, 2000

Regier DA, Burke JD: Epidemiology, in Kaplan and Sadock's Comprehensive Textbook of Psychiatry, 7th Edition. Edited by Sadock BJ, Sadock VA. Philadelphia, PA, Lippincott Williams & Wilkins, 2000, pp 500–522

Regier DA, Kaelber CT, Rae DS, et al: Limitations of diagnostic criteria and assessment instruments for mental disorders: implications for research and policy. Arch Gen Psychiatry 55:109–115, 1998

Robins LN: Birth and development of psychiatric interviews, in Textbook of Psychiatric Epidemiology, 2nd Edition. Edited by Tsuang MT, Tohen M. New York, Wiley-Liss, 2002, pp 257–271

Skodol AE, Bender DS: Diagnostic interviews for adults, in Handbook of Psychiatric Measures. Washington, DC, American Psychiatric Association, 2000, pp 45–70

Slater E, Cowie V: The Genetics of Mental Disorder. New York, Oxford University Press, 1971

Tsuang MT, Tohen M (eds): Textbook in Psychiatric Epidemiology, 2nd Edition. New York, Wiley-Liss, 2002

10

STUDIES OF RISK OR HARM

This chapter covers the appraisal of two types of studies: those that assess the *harm* associated with a therapy (e.g., medication side effects) and those that attempt to identify factors that increase the *risk* of developing a disease. A variety of study designs are presented, including case reports, randomized controlled trials (RCTs), cohort studies, and case-control studies (Levine et al. 2002; Turcotte et al. 2001) (Table 10–1).

■ CASE REPORTS AND CASE SERIES

As noted in Chapter 5, case reports and case series are best viewed as sources of hypotheses for further testing (Fletcher et al. 1996; Hennekens et al. 1987). They have been used traditionally to describe rare clinical events and often provide the first warnings about rare—but clinically significant—adverse drug reactions (ADRs) (Brewer and Colditz 1999).

Unfortunately, case reports and case series may also include coincidental occurrences, and without a denominator it is impossible to determine the actual risk of an adverse event. For example, case reports have wrongly implicated beta-blockers as a cause of depression, which actually occurs no more frequently in patients on beta-blockers than in patients receiving placebos (Ko et al. 2002).

■ RANDOMIZED CONTROLLED TRIALS

Although it would be unethical to conduct an RCT designed to cause harm to a subject, a considerable amount of information

TABLE 10–1.	Study designs used to assess etiology or harm			
	Case reports or case series	Randomized controlled trial (RCT)	Cohort study	Case-control study
Advantages	Used to describe rare or unusual events	Least biased study design Can demonstrate cause-effect relationship	Less apt to be biased than case-control study Better able to assess rare outcomes than RCT	Quicker, less expensive than cohort study Useful for rare diseases
Disadvantages	Cannot prove association or causality Often misleading	Cannot assess risk of rare side effects Unethical to conduct trial specifically to cause harm	Involves large numbers of subjects Loss to follow-up may limit validity	More prone to bias than RCT or cohort study Cannot measure absolute risks
Risk statistics	None	Relative risk increase Absolute risk increase Number needed to harm	Relative risk Risk difference Number needed to harm	Odds ratio

about common side effects of medications comes from Phase II and Phase III clinical trials (Jones 2001). Unfortunately, such reporting is often incomplete (Ioannidis and Lau 2001). Furthermore, pre-marketing trials are often of short duration, are limited to fewer than 2,000 patients, and simply do not have the statistical power to detect ADRs, which occur in 1 of 10,000 drug exposures (for which 30,000 patients would have to be studied) (Brewer and Colditz 1999; Pirmohamed et al. 1998).

For common side effects, however, an RCT provides the best evidence that the side effect was caused by medication, not chance (Turcotte et al. 2001) A variety of statistical measures are used to assess the magnitude of the difference in adverse events between a control and experimental treatments. Most of these measures are discussed in Chapter 5; however, there are three measures that are unique to studies of harm: relative risk increase (RRI), absolute risk increase (ARI), and number needed to harm (NNH) (Sackett et al. 2000) (Table 10–2).

Relative Risk and Relative Risk Increase

If a therapy increases the risk of an adverse event, the experimental event rate (EER) is greater than the control event rate (CER), and relative risk (RR), calculated as EER/CER, is greater than 1. RRI is calculated using the following formula:

$$RRI = \frac{EER - CER}{CER} = RR - 1$$

Because RR and RRI are relative measures, they do not provide an estimate of the actual increase in frequency of an adverse event. For example, an EER of 0.5% and a CER of 0.1% yield the same RR and RRI as an EER of 50% and an CER of 10%, yet the absolute magnitude of the increase in adverse events is greater in the latter case.

TABLE 10–2.   **Measures of risk: randomized controlled trial**

	Experimental treatment	**Control treatment**
Harm	A	B
No harm	C	D
Total	A+C	B+D

Experimental event rate (EER)=A/(A+C)
Control event rate (CER)=B/(B+D)
Relative risk (RR)=EER/CER
Relative risk increase=(EER−CER)/CER=RR−1
Absolute risk increase (ARI)=EER−CER
Number needed to harm=1/ARI

Absolute Risk Increase and Number Needed to Harm

ARI is calculated as EER−CER. Unlike RR and RRI, ARI provides a measure of the proportion of patients receiving treatment who will be harmed by it, which thus avoids some of the limitations of the relative measures of effect.

NNH is simply the reciprocal of ARI. It is analogous to NNT (see Chapter 5) as a measure of treatment effect; it indicates the number of patients who would need to be treated with the experimental treatment to produce one more adverse event than would have occurred with the control treatment.

■ EPIDEMIOLOGIC STUDIES

Because we do not ordinarily conduct experiments to prove that something is harmful to patients, much of our knowledge about the etiology of disease, as well as of less common medication side effects, comes from epidemiologic studies. In this section, the two most common study designs, cohort studies and case-control studies, are reviewed. The reader is referred to several excellent epidemiology texts for a more complete discussion (Fletcher et al. 1996; Gordis 2000; Hennekens et al. 1987; Kelsey et al. 1996; Rothman 2002).

Cohort Studies

In a cohort study, a group of subjects (cohort) is followed over time, and the incidence of disease is determined (see Chapter 9). The members of the cohort can be classified as either *exposed* or *unexposed* to a medication or suspected risk factor for disease. Such characteristics are determined at the beginning of the study, before disease occurrence. If exposure increases the risk of disease, the incidence in the exposed group is greater than the incidence in the unexposed group.

Prospective Cohort Studies

Cohort studies can be either prospective or retrospective (Hennekens et al. 1987). In a prospective or concurrent cohort study, the cohort is assembled and the exposure status is determined; it is then followed over time to determine the incidence of disease. In a prospective cohort study, Takeshita et al. (2002) followed a cohort of more than 3,000 Japanese Americans for 6 years and found that those with depressive symptoms had an increased mortality rate, compared with those without depressive symptoms.

Retrospective Cohort Studies

In a retrospective cohort study, existing records are used to identify an historical cohort and to measure both exposures and outcomes of interest, all of which have occurred at the time the study is initiated. Doing so allows the study to be conducted more quickly and with less expense than if the cohort was actually followed for several years. Because retrospective cohort studies are dependent on existing records, issues of data quality often arise. An example of a retrospective cohort study is that of Gunnell et al. (2002), in which intellectual performance at age 18 was determined from military psychological records for a cohort of nearly 200,000 Swedish male conscripts examined several years earlier and was found to predict the subsequent development of schizophrenia and other psychoses over an average follow-up period of 5 years.

Bias and Confounding

Cohort studies are sometimes referred to as *natural experiments*, although they differ significantly in that the subjects are not randomly allocated in a cohort study (Gordis 2000; Rothman 2002). This is an important difference, in that bias and confounding become major considerations in interpreting the results. In an RCT, randomization minimizes the chance that differences in outcomes between the experimental and control groups are the result of preexisting differences in the subjects in the two groups. In a cohort study, preexisting differences between exposed and nonexposed subjects may influence the subsequent risk of disease.

Confounding is especially problematic in studies of medication side effects, where the prescription of particular medications may be influenced by the preexisting medical conditions of patients, which is called *confounding by indication* (Rothman 2002). For example, because olanzapine causes more weight gain than risperidone (Lawrie and McIntosh 2002), risperidone might be prescribed more frequently to patients predisposed to obesity or diabetes, thus confounding any observed relationship between medication and risk of diabetes. Confounding can be accounted for in the statistical analysis of the data, but only to the extent that the confounding factors have been identified and measured. Statistical methods to control for confounding in cohort studies include stratified analysis and Poisson regression, details of which can be found in more advanced texts (Kelsey et al. 1996; Rothman and Greenland 1998).

There are also several potential biases in cohort studies that could be problematic. These include differential misclassification as to disease and exposure status, losses to follow-up, and nonparticipation. Good discussions of biases and confounding in cohort studies can be found in most standard epidemiology texts (Gordis 2000; Hennekens et al. 1987; Rothman 2002).

Measures of Risk

In a cohort study, incidence rates are calculated for exposed and nonexposed groups. Several measures of risk can then be calculated, including absolute risk, RR, odds ratio (OR), and risk difference (RD) (Table 10–3). RD in a cohort study is analogous to ARI in an RCT, and NNH may be calculated as 1/RD. RR and OR are measures of the strength of association between an exposure and outcome, whereas the RD and NNH are better measures of the potential for prevention (Gordis 2000; Sackett et al. 2000).

TABLE 10–3. **Measures of risk: cohort study**

	Exposed group	**Nonexposed group**
Harm	A	B
No harm	C	D
Total	A+C	B+D

Incidence in exposed group=A/(A+C)
Incidence in nonexposed group=B/(B+D)
Relative risk=incidence in exposed group/incidence in nonexposed group
Risk difference=incidence in exposed group−incidence in nonexposed group
Number needed to harm=1/RD

Case-Control Studies

The other major study design is the case-control study. In a case-control study, patients with a particular disease (cases) are compared with patients without the disease in question (i.e., controls) with regard to exposures and other characteristics. Case-control studies are especially useful in studying rare diseases, because cohort studies involve studying very large cohorts for extended periods of time for meaningful numbers of cases of rare diseases to occur.

By their nature, however, case-control studies are more susceptible to bias than are cohort studies and therefore rank lower on the hierarchy of evidence (Table 4–2, Chapter 4). Two of the major sources of bias relate to the choice of control subjects (selection bias) and the fact that information about exposure is gathered after the onset of disease (recall or information bias).

Choice of Controls

In a case-control study, control subjects must be chosen from the same source population as the cases, because control subjects are used to estimate the prevalence of exposure to a risk factor in the population from which the cases are drawn (Lewis and Pelosi 1990; Rothman 2002). In other words, if cases are identified from a particular clinic or hospital, control subjects must be individuals who similarly have obtained treatment from that same clinic or hospital if they have the disease in question. In many cases, there are multiple medical providers serving a geographic area; therefore, hypothetical source population is not defined by specific geographic boundaries, but rather by referral or care-seeking patterns.

Several potential sources of control subjects can be used, and each has its own advantages and limitations (Hennekens et al. 1987; Rothman 2002). Sources include general population controls, including those identified by random-digit dialing; hospital or clinic controls; and friends, relatives, or neighbors of the cases.

Although it is often convenient to draw control subjects from the same hospital or clinic as the cases, because they clearly come from the same source population, there are also some important limitations related to exposure status. In particular, hospitalized control subjects differ from individuals without disease in the frequency of exposures that are associated with the control subjects' own diseases. For example, if an investigator is interested in conducting a case-control study to determine if alcohol use is a risk factor for deliberate self-harm, it might be tempting to identify both cases and controls from hospital emergency room patients. Because alcohol use is also a risk factor for accidental injuries, violence, and a number of other diseases, obtaining control subjects from an emergency room overestimates the use of alcohol in the population without disease and hence tends to obscure any association with self-harm.

The "nested" case-control study, which minimizes some of the issues in control selection, is a variant of the case-control study (Gordis 2000; Rothman 2002). In a nested case-control study, both cases and controls come from a previously assembled cohort; therefore, there is an enumerated source population from which to select the controls. An example of a nested case-control study is that of Koro et al. (2002), in which cases of patients with diabetes and control subjects were obtained from a cohort of over 19,000 patients with schizophrenia who were in a general practice research database. The authors then assessed prior use of antipsychotic medication by the patients with diabetes and the control subjects and were able to demonstrate that olanzapine use increased the risk of developing diabetes.

Recall Bias

The other serious concern in case-control studies is recall bias. Individuals with a disease often search their memories for possible causes and are therefore more likely to selectively recall exposures than are control subjects; this is sometimes called *rumination bias* or *effort after meaning* (Creed 1993; Gordis 2000). In psychiatric epidemiology, there is the added problem that the psychiatric illness may selectively influence memory (Lewis and Pelosi 1990). For example, patients with depression are more apt to remember negative life experiences than are nondepressed individuals (Creed 1993; Lloyd and Lishman 1976).

Reverse Causality

An additional problem with case-control studies is that of reverse causality (Creed 1993; Lewis and Pelosi 1990). In a case-control study, cases are asked about exposures prior to the onset of illness. For some psychiatric illnesses, it is difficult to determine the exact onset of illness. In addition, it may be difficult to determine retrospectively if an event, such as marital discord, truly preceded the onset of illness or if it was a consequence of the illness. This has been a particular problem with life events and depression research (Cooper and Paykel 1993; Creed 1993).

Odds Ratio

The OR is the measure of risk in a case-control study (Table 10–4). For rare diseases, the OR approximates RR from a cohort study. Measures of absolute risk cannot be directly estimated from a case-control study. It is possible, however, to estimate NNH from the OR, if the incidence of disease in the unexposed population is known (Bjerre and LeLorier 2000). This method is described in Appendix B.

Causality in Epidemiologic Studies

There are several explanations for an association between an exposure and a disease in an epidemiologic study (Table 10–5), including bias, chance, confounding, and causality (Fletcher et al. 1996; Hennekens et al. 1987).

TABLE 10–4. **Measure of risk: case-control study**

	Cases	Controls
Exposed	A	B
Nonexposed	C	D

Odds ratio=(A/C)/(B/D)=(AD)/(BC)

TABLE 10–5. **Explanations for associations between exposure and disease in epidemiologic studies**

Bias
Selection bias
Information bias

Chance

Confounding

Causality

Bias

Bias refers to a systematic error that results in an incorrect estimate of the risk of disease associated with an exposure. Bias may occur as a result of the process of selecting subjects (selection bias) or from gathering information on exposures (information or recall bias). As noted above, case-control studies are more susceptible to selection and information biases than are prospective cohort studies.

Chance

Chance is always a possible explanation for an observed association between an exposure and a disease. The likelihood that chance alone is responsible is assessed through tests of statistical significance (*P* values) and confidence intervals (see Chapter 5).

Confounding

Confounding involves the possibility that differences in subjects (other than the exposure under investigation) are responsible for the observed association between the exposure and the disease. For example, if women in a retirement community are, on average, older than men, an observed increased risk of Alzheimer's disease in women could be the result of an association with age rather than with female sex. In other words, age is a confounding factor. If there are potential confounding factors that have been measured in a study, the statistical analysis of the data can take them into account, either through stratified analysis or regression techniques (i.e., Poisson regression for a cohort study or logistic regression for a case-control study) (Kelsey et al. 1996; Rothman and Greenland 1998).

Causality

If bias, chance, and confounding are not the explanations for an association between exposure and disease, a causal relationship is likely.

Bradford Hill (1965) described a variety of evidence that would support a causal relationship. Table 10–6 presents some of the criteria for causation suggested by Bradford Hill (1965) and others (Elwood 1998; Fletcher et al. 1996; Gordis 2000; Hennekens et al. 1987; Turcotte et al. 2001). Although Rothman (2002) has criticized such "checklists" as not reflecting more sophisticated notions of causality, many other epidemiologists continue to find them useful.

■ CRITICAL APPRAISAL GUIDES FOR STUDIES OF ETIOLOGY OR HARM

Tables 10–7 through 10–9 are the critical appraisal guides for studies of etiology or harm. Separate guides are provided for RCT, cohort study, and case-control study, the three major study designs.

■ RANDOMIZED CONTROLLED TRIAL REPORTING HARM

Is the Study Valid?

Before reviewing the results of the RCT, you should first ensure that the study is valid. The criteria for doing this are similar to those for appraising studies designed to evaluate the efficacy of a therapy (Table 5–6, Chapter 5). However, there are some additional considerations for a study of adverse effects.

First, were the adverse effects assessed in a systematic way (as opposed to self reporting)? Some side effects (e.g., sexual side effects) may not be spontaneously reported because of embarrassment. Not asking about a specific side effect may lead to misleadingly low rates.

Second, was the size of the study sufficient to detect meaningful differences in rates of the side effects of interest? RCTs lack sufficient power to detect rare side effects; however, if a particular side effect (e.g., weight gain) is of interest, the study should have sufficient power to detect meaningful differences.

TABLE 10-6. **Suggested criteria for causality in epidemiologic studies**

Criterion	Description
Temporal relationship	Exposure precedes disease
Strength of association	Large relative risk or odds ratio
Dose–response relationship	Increasing exposure increases risk
Reversibility	Reducing exposure decreases risk
Consistency	Similar findings from other studies in different populations
Biological plausibility	Consistent with pharmacological or toxicological data
Analogy	Relationship established for similar cause and disease
Elimination of other explanations	Not the result of confounding or bias
Specificity	One cause, one effect

Source. Adapted from Fletcher et al. 1996; Gordis 2000; Hennekens et al. 1987; Sackett et al. 2000.

TABLE 10–7.   **Critical appraisal guide for randomized controlled trials reporting harm**

Is the study valid?

Is it a randomized controlled trial?

Was the randomization list concealed?

Were subjects and clinicians blinded to treatment being administered?

Were side effects assessed appropriately?

Was the trial of sufficient duration to detect the side effects of interest?

Were all subjects enrolled in the trial accounted for?

Were subjects analyzed in the groups to which they were assigned?

Despite randomization, were there clinically important differences between groups at the start of the trial?

Aside from the experimental treatment, were the groups treated equally?

Are the results important?

How large was the treatment effect (number needed to harm)?

How precise are the results (width of confidence intervals)?

Can I apply the results to my patient?

Is my patient too different from patients in the study?

How do the benefits and risks of treatment compare for my patient?

How does my patient value these benefits and risks?

Do the benefits outweigh the harms (likelihood of being helped or harmed)?

Source.   Based in part on the criteria of Levine et al. 2002; Sackett et al. 2000.

Are the Results Important?

In an RCT that reports adverse effects, NNH is the measure of interest. In addition, the severity of side effects, not only the frequency, is important.

Can I Apply the Results to My Patient?

As noted in Chapter 5, this question can be reframed as: "Is the biology of my patient so different from that of the study patients that the results cannot apply?" Here the considerations regarding side effects become more complicated than with the assessment of beneficial effects. There are often significant differences in the risk of adverse effects, depending on patient characteristics. To take an obvious example, men and nonpregnant women are not at risk for the teratogenic side effects of a medication. Beyond this, however, there are a variety of physical illnesses that could be exacerbated by a medication or that could predispose a patient to a particular side effect. In addition, there are age-related changes in drug metabolism, and members of particular ethnic groups may be at increased risk of specific medication side effects, partly because of allelic variation in genes coding for drug-metabolizing enzymes (Cookson et al. 2002; Ruiz 2000). Thus, some judgment is required in deciding whether your patient is enough like those in the study that the results apply and whether your patient is at increased or decreased risk. In general, your patient will probably be similar enough to those studied that the results will apply, although the magnitude of the risk may differ.

In assessing the relative risks and benefits of treatment, the issue is one of comparing NNT as a measure of treatment effectiveness with NNH as a measure of treatment side effects. This can certainly be done informally by simply comparing NNT and NNH, together with a subjective assessment of the relative value the patient places on the benefit versus the risk. A more formal quantitative method of doing this has been described that involves calculating a statistic, the likelihood of being helped or harmed (LHH) (Guyatt et al. 2002; Sackett et al. 2000). As a first approximation:

$$LHH = \frac{1/NNT}{1/NNH} = \frac{NNH}{NNT}$$

with values of LHH>1 indicating that the benefit outweighs the harm. This crude calculation weights benefits and side effects equally. A more sophisticated calculation, taking into account patients' relative preferences for side effects versus treatment effects, (as well as patient-specific NNTs and NNHs) is given in Appendix B.

■ COHORT STUDIES OF ETIOLOGY OR HARM

A critical appraisal guide for a cohort study of etiology or harm is given in Table 10–8.

Is the Study Valid?

Several questions should be asked to determine the validity of the study. First, how were the subjects selected? The cohort should consist of individuals who are initially free of the disease under investigation, but who are potentially at risk for developing the disease. In addition, the exposed and nonexposed groups should be selected in such a way as to avoid major differences other than exposure status.

TABLE 10–8.   **Critical appraisal guide for cohort studies**

Is the study valid?

Were the exposed and nonexposed groups similar (other than exposure) to the risk factor at the onset of the study?

If there were differences between groups at the start of the trial, did the statistical analysis take the differences into account?

Was the follow-up of the cohort sufficiently long for outcomes to develop?

Were outcomes measured in the same way in both groups?

Were there significant differences in losses to follow-up in the two groups?

Were any of the criteria for causality met (Table 10–6)?

Are the results important?

How strong is the association (relative risk)?

How large is the absolute increase in risk (risk difference)?

Can I apply the results to my patient?

Is my patient too different from patients in the study?

How do the benefits and risks of treatment compare for my patient?

How does my patient value these benefits and risks?

Do the benefits outweigh the harms (likelihood of being helped or harmed)?

Source.   Based in part on the criteria of Elwood 1998; Levine et al. 2002; Sackett et al. 2000.

Was the cohort large enough and was the follow-up period long enough? For rare outcomes, large numbers of individuals must often be studied for prolonged periods of time to detect statistically significant differences in risk.

How was exposure measured? If significant errors are made in classifying individuals as either "exposed" or not, the results will tend to be biased. Random misclassification will tend to bias the observed RR toward 1.0, whereas differential misclassification will result in either an overestimate or underestimate of the actual RR (Hennekens et al. 1987).

Were exposed and unexposed individuals assessed for outcomes with the same intensity and were outcomes assessed blindly (i.e., without knowledge of exposure status)? If not, any differences could be the result of measurement bias, not true differences (Fletcher et al. 1996).

Similarly, were there differences in dropout rates between the two groups? Because the outcomes of patients who drop out may differ from the outcomes of patients completing the study, differences in dropout rates between the two groups may lead to biased estimates of risk (Hennekens et al. 1987).

Were the exposed and nonexposed groups in fact similar, except for exposure? If not, then confounding may be responsible for any difference in risk that is observed. If there were differences in potential confounding factors, appropriate statistical techniques (stratification or multivariate techniques) should have been used in the data analysis.

Were any of the criteria for causality (Table 10–6) met? If so, the likelihood that the results were not the result of chance, bias, or confounding is increased.

Are the Results Important?

In a cohort study, RR measures the strength of association between the exposure and outcome, whereas NNH is a better measure of the potential harm to an individual patient (Sackett et al. 2000).

Can I Apply the Results to My Patient?

As with RCTs, this question can be reframed in the following way: "Is the biology of my patient so different from that of the study patients that the results cannot apply?"

If the clinical question is one that concerns the etiology of a disorder, the results will generally be applicable, assuming that your patient could be at risk for the outcome and bearing in mind that some outcomes are limited to patients who are of a particular age, sex, or childbearing status. With regard to etiology, the assumptions are that RR will apply to all individuals and that risks are generally multiplicative. In certain circumstances, however, interactions between risk factors that could either increase or decrease a particular patient's risk beyond what is expected by the RR associated with the individual risk factors are possible (Gordis 2000; Rothman 2002).

In assessing the absolute risk to an individual patient, however, NNH is used as the measure of risk. Unlike RR, this measure is sensitive to the individual's baseline risk and may need to be individualized.

As with an RCT, in assessing the relative risks and benefits of treatment, the issue is one of comparing NNT (usually derived from an RCT) with NNH from the cohort study, and the same considerations apply as discussed for LHH above.

■ CASE-CONTROL STUDY

A critical appraisal guide for a case-control study is given in Table 10–9.

Is the Study Valid?

The first question is how the cases were chosen. The cases should be representative of patients with the disease. In addition, they should be incident (newly diagnosed) cases, because a study of prevalent cases may reveal more about risk factors for chronicity than about the etiology of the disorder.

TABLE 10–9.	Critical appraisal guide for case-control studies

Is the study valid?

Did the method of selection of cases and control subjects introduce bias?

Were outcomes measured in the same way in both groups, independent of disease status?

Were confounding factors identified and dealt with in the analysis?

Were any of the criteria for causality met (Table 10–6)?

Are the results important?

How strong is the association (odds ratio)?

Can I apply the results to my patient?

Is my patient too different from patients in the study?

What is the number needed to harm for my patient?

How do the benefits and risks of treatment compare for my patient?

How does my patient value these benefits and risks?

Do the benefits outweigh the harms (likelihood of being helped or harmed)?

Source. Based in part on the criteria of Fletcher et al. 1996; Levine et al. 2002; Mant 1999; Sackett et al. 2000.

The next question is how the control subjects were chosen. In a case-control study, control subjects must be chosen from the same source population as the cases, because control subjects are used to estimate the prevalence of exposure to a risk factor in the population from which the cases are drawn (Lewis and Pelosi 1990; Rothman 2002). In other words, if the cases in a study were identified from a particular clinic or hospital, would the control subjects have obtained treatment from that same clinic or hospital if they had the disease in question? Control subjects can include general population controls; hospital or clinic controls; and friends, relatives, or neighbors of the cases. If more than one control group was used in a particular study, were the results similar? If so, it is less likely that the results were the result of selection bias.

The other serious concern in case-control studies is information or recall bias. Exposure history should be gathered without knowledge of whether the individual is a case or a control subject.

In addition, using more than one information source may increase the validity of the information being collected, because individuals with a disease often search their memories for possible causes, and psychiatric illnesses may selectively influence memory.

Were the cases and the control subjects generally similar except for exposure? If not, confounding may be responsible for any difference in the amount of risk that is observed. If there were differences in potential confounding factors, appropriate statistical techniques (stratification or multivariate techniques) should have been used in the data analysis.

Were any of the criteria for causality (Table 10–6) met? If so, the likelihood that the results were not the result of chance, bias, or confounding is increased.

Are the Results Important?

In a case-control study, the OR measures the strength of association between the exposure and the outcome. Measures of absolute risk cannot be determined from a case-control study alone.

Can I Apply the Results to My Patient?

As in a cohort study, if the clinical question concerns the etiology of a disorder, the results will generally be applicable, assuming your patient could be at risk for the outcome. The assumptions are that the OR will apply to all individuals and that risks are multiplicative. There may be interactions between risk factors that may either increase or decrease a particular patient's risk beyond what would be expected from the OR associated with the individual risk factors (Gordis 2000; Rothman 2002).

Because measures of absolute risk cannot be directly estimated from a case-control study, the study itself will not yield NNH. It is possible, however, to estimate NNH from the OR if the probability of disease in the patient (usually estimated from the incidence of disease in the population) is known (Bjerre and LeLorier 2000). A method for calculating this estimation is given in Appendix B. As in an RCT or cohort study, the issue in assessing the relative risks and benefits of treatment becomes one of comparing NNT (usually derived from an RCT) with NNH (estimated from the OR and population incidence data).

■ REFERENCES

Bjerre LM, LeLorier J: Expressing the magnitude of adverse effects in case-control studies: "the number of patients needed to be treated for one additional patient to be harmed." BMJ 320:503–506, 2000

Bradford Hill AB: The environment and disease: association and causation. Proc R Soc Med 58:295–300, 1965

Brewer T, Colditz GA: Postmarketing surveillance and adverse drug reactions: current perspectives and future needs. JAMA 281:824–829, 1999

Cookson J, Taylor D, Katona C: The Use of Drugs in Psychiatry: The Evidence from Psychopharmacology, 5th Edition. London, Gaskell, 2002

Cooper Z, Paykel ES: Social factors in the onset and maintenance of depression, in Principles of Social Psychiatry. Edited by Bhugra D, Leff J. London, Blackwell Scientific, 1993, pp 99–121

Creed F: Life events, in Principles of Social Psychiatry. Edited by Bhugra D, Leff J. London, Blackwell Scientific, 1993, pp 144–161

Elwood M: Critical Appraisal of Epidemiological Studies and Clinical Trials, 2nd Edition. Oxford, Oxford University Press, 1998

Fletcher RH, Fletcher SW, Wagner EH: Clinical Epidemiology: The Essentials, 3rd Edition. Baltimore, MD, Williams & Wilkins, 1996

Gordis L: Epidemiology, 2nd Edition. Philadelphia, PA, WB Saunders, 2000

Gunnell D, Harrison G, Rasmussen F, et al: Associations between premorbid intellectual performance, early life exposures and early onset schizophrenia: cohort study. Br J Psychiatry 181:298–305, 2002

Guyatt G, Straus S, McAlister F, et al: Moving from evidence to action: incorporating patient values, in Users' Guides to the Medical Literature: A Manual for Evidence-Based Clinical Practice. Edited by Guyatt G, Rennie D. Chicago, IL, AMA Press, 2002, pp 567–582

Hennekens CH, Buring JE, Mayrent SL: Epidemiology in Medicine. Boston, MA, Little, Brown, 1987

Ioannidis JPA, Lau J: Completeness of safety reporting in randomized trials: an evaluation of 7 medical areas. JAMA 285:437–443, 2001

Jones TC: Call for a new approach to the process of clinical trials and drug registration. BMJ 322:920–923, 2001

Kelsey JL, Whittemore AS, Evans AS, et al (eds): Methods in Observational Epidemiology, 2nd Edition. New York, Oxford University Press, 1996

Ko DT, Hebert PR, Coffey CS, et al: Beta-blocker therapy and symptoms of depression, fatigue, and sexual dysfunction. JAMA 288:351–357, 2002

Koro CE, Fedder DO, L'Italien GJ, et al: Assessment of independent effect of olanzapine and risperidone on risk of diabetes among patients with schizophrenia: population based nested case-control study. BMJ 325:243–245, 2002

Lawrie S, McIntosh A: Schizophrenia. Clin Evid 7:920–944, 2002

Levine M, Haslam D, Walter S, et al: Harm, in Users' Guides to the Medical Literature: A Manual for Evidence-Based Clinical Practice. Edited by Guyatt G, Rennie D. Chicago, IL, AMA Press, 2002, pp 81–100

Lewis G, Pelosi AJ: The case-control study in psychiatry. Br J Psychiatry 157:197–207, 1990

Lloyd G, Lishman A: The effect of depression on speed of recall of pleasant and unpleasant experiences. Psychol Med 5:173–190, 1976

Mant J: Case-control studies, in Evidence-Based Practice: A Primer for Health Care Professionals. Edited by Dawes M, Davies P, Gray A, et al. Edinburgh, Churchill Livingstone, 1999, pp 73–84

Pirmohamed M, Breckenridge AM, Kitteringham NR, et al: Adverse drug reactions. BMJ 316:1295–1298, 1998

Rothman KJ: Epidemiology: An Introduction. New York, Oxford University Press, 2002

Rothman KJ, Greenland S (eds): Modern Epidemiology, 2nd Edition. Philadelphia, PA, Lippincott-Raven, 1998

Ruiz P (ed): Ethnicity and Psychopharmacology (Review of Psychiatry Series, Vol 19, No 4). Washington, DC, American Psychiatric Press, 2000

Sackett DL, Strauss SE, Richardson WS, et al: Evidence-Based Medicine: How to Practice and Teach EBM, 2nd Edition. New York, Churchill Livingstone, 2000

Takeshita J, Masaki K, Ahmed I, et al: Are depressive symptoms a risk factor for mortality in elderly Japanese American men? The Honolulu-Asia Aging Study. Am J Psychiatry 159:1127–1132, 2002

Turcotte K, Raina P, Moyer VA: Above all, do no harm. West J Med 174: 325–329, 2001

11

STUDIES OF PROGNOSIS

Questions about prognosis are frequently raised by patients and by their families. Such questions take many forms. When will I get better? Will I be completely well? What are the chances of the disease recurring? Such questions are studied by following groups of patients over time (i.e., in a cohort study). Some such studies are purely descriptive, whereas other studies attempt to find prognostic factors that predict a good or bad outcome. The latter types are similar to the cohort studies of risk described in Chapter 10 and are subject to the same design and analysis issues. This chapter focuses on descriptive studies of prognosis and briefly reviews some of the issues in their design and analysis before discussing their critical appraisal.

■ SELECTING PATIENTS

The selection of patients in a cohort study of prognosis is of considerable importance. The two key issues are the populations from which the subjects are obtained and whether they are newly diagnosed cases or patients currently in treatment.

Source of Patients

One can think of several populations of patients with the same illness: patients in the general population who are in treatment with non–mental health practitioners, those in outpatient treatment with mental health professionals, those in specialized mental health clinics (e.g., an academic mood disorders clinic), and those who are hospitalized for their conditions. In general, patients seen at academic medical centers have more severe disease, more comorbid conditions, and are more likely to be treatment resistant or chronically ill than are those in community settings (Cohen and Cohen 1984; Hulley et al. 2001; Randolph et al. 2002). We know far less about the prognosis of individuals in the community who do not seek treatment (Regier et al. 1998), but it is believed that they have a better prognosis and more social supports (Cohen and Cohen 1984).

An example of such a difference in prognosis comes from a study of the duration of major depressive episodes in the general population conducted by Spijker et al. (2002). In this study, cases were identified as part of a prospective epidemiological study in a community, so the authors were able to identify cases that did not seek treatment, as well as those that did. Median durations of the depressive episode were 3.0 months for patients who had no professional care, 4.5 months for patients treated in primary care settings, and 6.0 months for patients who entered the mental health system.

There is no "right" population to study, but the population studied affects the generalizability of the results (Gordis 2000; Randolph et al. 2002). Results obtained from a study of patients in an academic medical center may not apply to individuals in the community.

Incident Versus Prevalent Cases

The other major issue concerns whether to select new (incident) cases or existing (prevalent) cases. There is a temptation to begin with a cohort of patients already in treatment (a survival cohort), but such a sample would contain an overrepresentation of chronic patients and hence lead to a biased estimate of prognosis (Cohen and Cohen 1984; Fletcher et al. 1996). Instead, an inception cohort (a group of people assembled near the onset of disease) should be studied (Fletcher et al. 1996).

A related issue is that of the starting point or *zero time*

(Fletcher et al. 1996; Gordis 2000). This could either be at the onset of symptoms, when treatment was first begun, or when a diagnosis was made. Regardless of what is chosen as the zero time, it should be used consistently as the starting point (Fletcher et al. 1996).

■ FOLLOW-UP AND ATTRITION

One of the major sources of bias in cohort studies of prognosis concerns patients lost to follow-up. If patients lost to follow-up differ in outcomes from patients who remain in the study, estimates of prognosis will be biased. This is called *migration bias* (Fletcher et al. 1996).

One way of dealing with losses to follow-up in the analysis is to perform a *best case/worst case* analysis, a form of sensitivity analysis in which outcome statistics are first calculated assuming all of those lost to follow-up did well, then recalculated assuming all of those lost to follow-up had a bad outcome (Fletcher et al. 1996; Sackett et al. 2000). Ideally, researchers should attempt to minimize losses to follow-up through periodic contact and other means (Cummings et al. 2001).

■ OUTCOMES AND DATA ANALYSIS

There are two commonly used approaches for describing the prognosis of a cohort: reporting on outcomes at specified follow-up times and measuring time to an event.

Outcomes at Specific Follow-Up Times

Investigators will sometimes recontact a cohort at specified times and collect data for a variety of outcome measures. Such an approach was taken by Wiersma et al. (2000) when they used several measures of social disability to assess a cohort of patients with schizophrenia at 1, 2, and 15 years after diagnosis. The advantage of this approach is that considerable information can be collected at each follow-up interview. The disadvantage is that no information is gathered between the set follow-up intervals, and the losses that follow lead to data that are based on smaller and smaller numbers of subjects at each subsequent interview.

Time-to-Event Outcomes: Survival Analysis

The use of time-to-event as an outcome measure in studies of prognosis is more common than the use of specified follow-up times. The event may be a negative one (e.g., death, relapse, rehospitalization, or dropping out of treatment) or a positive one (e.g., recovery). Such data are analyzed using statistical techniques called *survival analysis* or *failure time analysis*.

Survival analysis acknowledges that patients may be lost to follow-up; however, the analysis does include these patients until such time as they are lost. A basic statistical assumption, however, is that the prognosis of patients lost to follow-up (i.e., censored) will be the same as for patients who continue in the study (Bland and Altman 1998; Gordis 2000). Survival curves, such as the one in Figure 11–1, are calculated using the Kaplan-Meier method, the details of which are given in standard biostatistics texts (e.g., Altman 1991; Pagano and Gauvreau 2000). The log-rank test can be used to test for differences in survival times between subgroups (Altman 1991; Peto et al. 1977).

■ CRITICAL APPRAISAL GUIDE FOR STUDIES OF PROGNOSIS

Guidelines for appraising cohort studies of prognosis are given in Table 11–1. As with other types of studies, validity should be assessed before considering the results.

Is the Study Valid?

The study should be based on an inception (incidence) cohort. If it is based on a survival cohort of patients at various stages of illness,

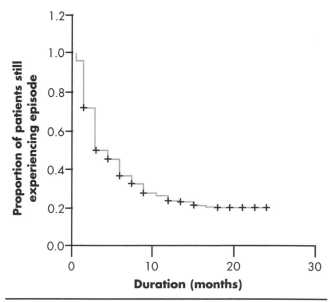

FIGURE 11–1. **Survival curve of a cohort with newly originated major depression in the community.**

Source. Reprinted from Spijker J, DeGraaf R, Bijl RV, et al: "Duration of Major Depressive Episodes in the General Population: Results From The Netherlands Mental Health Survey and Incidence Study (NEMESIS)." *British Journal of Psychiatry* 181:208–213, 2002. Copyright 2002 Royal College of Psychiatrists. Used with permission.

it is simply not a valid study of prognosis.

The next question concerns follow-up losses. Sackett et al. (2000) have suggested using the "5 and 20" guideline, where <5% of patients lost to follow-up is probably not significant, whereas >20% lost to follow-up seriously threatens the validity of the study.

Finally, it is important that study outcomes be assessed in a uniform way.

TABLE 11–1.	**Critical appraisal guide for studies of prognosis**

Is the study valid?
Is it a cohort study based on an inception cohort?
Was the follow-up relatively complete (>80% and preferably >95%)?
Were outcomes assessed in a uniform, unbiased manner?

What are the results?
What are the outcome data at various points in time?
Is there a survival curve?
How precise are the estimates?

Can I apply the results to my patient?
Were the patients similar to my patients in diagnosis and comorbidity?
Were the patients derived from a similar treatment setting?
Was the management similar to that in my practice?

Source. Based in part on data from Randolph et al. 2002; Sackett et al. 2000.

What Are the Results?

If measures other than time-to-event data are used, results should be presented with confidence intervals. Time-to-event data are generally presented in the form of a survival curve, often omitting confidence intervals for the curve itself but providing some information in the text on precision of the estimates.

Can I Apply the Results to My Patient?

As noted above, the prognosis of a community sample may differ significantly from that obtained from various treatment settings. Whenever possible, an attempt should be made to find a study reporting on a population from a setting similar to that of your patient. If this is not possible, the results may still be usable, keeping in mind the general rule that cohorts assembled from an academic medical center or specialty mental health program will often contain a greater number of poor-prognosis patients than will cohorts assembled from primary care or community settings.

A secondary consideration has to do with comorbidity and

other patient attributes that may affect prognosis. Again, there are no hard and fast rules, but patients with comorbid conditions frequently have a worse prognosis than do patients without comorbid conditions. Once again, although this does not invalidate a study, some mental adjustment of the results must be made in applying them to your patient.

■ REFERENCES

Altman DG: Practical Statistics for Medical Research. Boca Raton, FL, Chapman and Hall, 1991

Bland JM, Altman DG: Survival probabilities (the Kaplan-Meier method). BMJ 317:1572, 1998

Cohen P, Cohen J: The clinician's illusion. Arch Gen Psychiatry 41:1178–1182, 1984

Cummings SR, Newman TB, Hulley SB: Designing an observational study: cohort studies, in Designing Clinical Research: An Epidemiologic Approach, 2nd Edition. Philadelphia, PA, Lippincott Williams and Wilkins, 2001, pp 95–105

Fletcher RH, Fletcher SW, Wagner EH: Clinical Epidemiology: The Essentials, 3rd Edition. Baltimore, MD, Williams & Wilkins, 1996

Gordis L: Epidemiology, 2nd Edition. Philadelphia, PA, WB Saunders, 2000

Hulley SB, Newman TB, Cummings SR: Choosing the study subjects: specification, sampling, and recruitment, in Designing Clinical Research: An Epidemiologic Approach, 2nd Edition. Philadelphia, PA, Lippincott Williams and Wilkins, 2001, pp 25–35

Pagano M, Gauvreau K: Principles of Biostatistics, 2nd Edition. Pacific Grove, CA, Duxbury, 2000

Peto R, Pike MC, Armitage P, et al: Design and analysis of randomized clinical trials requiring prolonged observation of each patient, II: analysis and examples. Br J Cancer 35:1–39, 1977

Randolph A, Bucher H, Richardson WS, et al: Prognosis, in Users' Guides to the Medical Literature: A Manual for Evidence-Based Clinical Care. Edited by Guyatt G, Rennie D. Chicago, IL, AMA Press, 2002, pp 141–154

Regier DA, Kaelber CT, Rae DS, et al: Limitations of diagnostic criteria and assessment instruments for mental disorders: implications for research and policy. Arch Gen Psychiatry 55:109–115, 1998

Sackett DL, Strauss SE, Richardson WS, et al: Evidence-Based Medicine: How to Practice and Teach EBM, 2nd Edition. New York, Churchill Livingstone, 2000

Spijker J, DeGraaf R, Bijl RV, et al: Duration of major depressive episodes in the general population: results from The Netherlands Mental Health Survey and Incidence Study (NEMESIS). Br J Psychiatry 181:208–213, 2002

Wiersma D, Wanderling J, Dragomirecka E, et al: Social disability in schizophrenia: its development and prediction over 15 years in incidence cohorts in six European cities. Psychol Med 30:1155–1167, 2000

12

EVALUATING YOUR
PERFORMANCE

In the 5-step evidence-based medicine (EBM) model (see Chapter 2), the final step is assessing the outcome. In ordinary clinical practice, we assess whether a particular treatment worked or whether a diagnostic test provided helpful information. In the EBM model, assessment has the added component of evaluating the clinician's performance in the EBM process.

The model for such an evaluation, as suggested by Sackett et al. (2000) and Wolf (2000), focuses on skills in performing each of the five steps in the EBM process (Table 12–1). A more in-depth discussion of the evaluation of clinical skills in general—and of EBM skills in particular—can be found in the works of Sackett et al. (1991, 2000).

■ FORMULATING CLINICAL QUESTIONS

The first necessary skill is formulating the 4-part clinical questions (see Chapter 3). Such a skill is important because it leads to a more efficient search strategy (Cabell et al. 2001), yet it is still one with which physicians may have difficulty (Ely et al. 2002).

The first question to ask is whether you understand the concept of the 4-part PICO clinical question (i.e., patient/problem, intervention, comparison, and outcome, as described in Chapter 3) and whether you were able to formulate such questions before beginning your most recent search for information. The next question to

TABLE 12–1. **Self-evaluation of evidence-based medicine skills**

Formulating clinical questions

Do I understand what a 4-part PICO clinical question is?

Was I able to formulate a 4-part PICO question this time?

Do I routinely keep track of clinical questions that arise in my practice and attempt to find answers to them?

Searching for answers

Do I know the common databases and how to search them?

Did this particular search go well or could I have been more efficient?

Do I routinely attempt to answer clinical questions through searches or do I still rely primarily on textbooks?

Appraising the evidence

Do I understand how to critically appraise research articles and other evidence?

Was I able to apply the critical appraisal guide in this case, including considering my patient's individual risks, needs, and preferences?

Are my critical appraisal skills improving over time?

Applying the evidence

Do I incorporate the evidence that I have appraised (and have found to be valid) into my clinical practice?

What proportion of my clinical decisions is based on current best evidence?

Evaluating the results

Do I routinely evaluate my evidence-based medicine skills?

Are there particular aspects of the evidence-based medicine process that I need to review?

Note.   PICO=patient/problem, intervention, comparison, and outcome.

ask is whether you routinely formulate such questions in your clinical practice.

Clinical questions arise every day in clinical practice, but we often do not have the ability to answer them on the spot (Del Mar and Glasziou 2001). To incorporate EBM into daily practice requires that we have a way of keeping track of the most important questions so that they can be answered at a later time.

■ SEARCHING FOR ANSWERS

The next step in the process is searching for an answer to the clinical question. In evaluating a particular search, barriers to finding the information should be identified. Common barriers include lack of time and information resources, as well as the search strategy itself (Cabell et al. 2001; Craig et al. 2001; Ely et al. 2002; McColl et al. 1998). Furthermore, many practitioners either lack awareness of the *Cochrane Database* and other resources or they do not use them, even if available (Kerse et al. 2001; McColl et al. 1998).

In evaluating your own performance, the first question to ask is whether you have an understanding of the basic search process (as outlined in Chapter 4), including the roles of the various databases that are available. The second question relates to your ability to perform the particular search and whether another search strategy would have proved more efficient. The final question to ask is whether you are routinely searching for answers using appropriate databases in your clinical practice, rather than relying on textbooks.

■ APPRAISING THE EVIDENCE

Critical appraisal skills are the most commonly taught aspect of EBM (Green 1999), yet clinicians often remain unfamiliar with many of the basic concepts (LeClair et al. 1999; McColl et al. 1998; Young et al. 2002). Such skills, however, are associated with the ability and willingness to apply the results of systematic reviews in clinical practice (Doust and Silagy 2000).

In evaluating yourself, the first question to ask is whether you have an understanding of the methods of critical appraisal, including the use of critical appraisal worksheets. (To review this information, see Chapters 5–11.) The next question to ask is whether you had any difficulties in appraising the evidence from this particular search. This also involves considering whether the evidence was applicable to your patient, being able to individualize the results for your patient, and assessing whether it was consistent with patient needs and preferences. Finally, you should ask whether your appraisal skills are improving over time as a result of practice.

■ APPLYING THE EVIDENCE

The fourth step involves applying the evidence to a particular patient. This is the step where we often falter (Wolf 2000). The most important question to ask here is whether your practice is becoming more evidence based. This can be done informally—for example, as you see patients, ask yourself whether the treatment provided, diagnostic test ordered, and so forth is supported by good evidence. This may encourage you to conduct searches for some common treatments that you are using, and the results may surprise you. It can also be done in a more formal way, as part of a quality improvement project (Baker and Grol 2001).

■ EVALUATING THE RESULTS

Finally, reflect on your own performance. How are you doing with your practice of EBM? If you are having problems with particular aspects, you may wish to review Chapter 13, which describes a number of resources for improving your EBM skills. Remember that your skill in practicing EBM is like any other skill: it gets easier with practice.

■ REFERENCES

Baker R, Grol R: How to assess the effectiveness of applying the evidence, in Evidence-Based Practice in Primary Care, 2nd Edition. Edited by Silagy C, Haines A. London, BMJ Books, 2001, pp 83–97

Cabell CH, Schardt C, Sanders L, et al: Resident utilization of information technology: a randomized trial of clinical question formation. J Gen Intern Med 16:838–844, 2001

Craig JC, Irwig LM, Stockler MR: Evidence-based medicine: useful tools for decision making. Med J Aust 174:248–253, 2001

Del Mar CB, Glasziou PP: Ways of using evidence-based medicine in general practice. Med J Aust 174:347–350, 2001

Doust JA, Silagy CA: Applying the results of a systematic review in general practice. Med J Aust 172:153–156, 2000

Ely JW, Osheroff JA, Ebell MH, et al: Obstacles to answering doctors' questions about patient care with evidence: qualitative study. BMJ 324:710–713, 2002

Green ML: Graduate medical education training in clinical epidemiology, critical appraisal, and evidence-based medicine: a critical review of the curricula. Acad Med 74:686–694, 1999

Kerse N, Arroll B, Lloyd T, et al: Evidence databases, the Internet, and general practitioners: the New Zealand story. N Z Med J 114:89–91, 2001

LeClair BM, Wagner PJ, Miller MD: A tool to evaluate self-efficacy in evidence-based medicine. Acad Med 74:597, 1999

McColl A, Smith H, White P, et al: General practitioners' perceptions of the route to evidence based medicine: a questionnaire survey. BMJ 316:361–365, 1998

Sackett DL, Haynes RB, Guyatt GH, et al: Clinical Epidemiology: A Basic Science for Clinical Medicine, 2nd Edition. Boston, MA, Little, Brown, 1991

Sackett DL, Straus SE, Richardson WS, et al: Evidence-Based Medicine: How to Practice and Teach EBM, 2nd Edition. New York, Churchill Livingstone, 2000

Wolf FM: Lessons to be learned from evidence-based medicine: practice and promise of evidence-based medicine and evidence-based education. Med Teach 22:251–259, 2000

Young JM, Glasziou P, Ward JE: General practitioners' self ratings of skills in evidence based medicine: validation study. BMJ 324:950–951, 2002

LEARNING AND PRACTICING EVIDENCE-BASED PSYCHIATRY

Surveys of physicians have consistently identified three factors that interfere with the application of the evidence-based medicine (EBM) model in everyday clinical practice: lack of time, lack of access to information resources, and lack of skill and knowledge (Craig et al. 2001; Ely et al. 2002; Geddes and Carney 2001; McColl et al. 1998; Young and Ward 2001). This chapter addresses these and other barriers to the incorporation of EBM into psychiatric practice.

■ INCREASING KNOWLEDGE AND SKILL

There are a number of routes that can be used to increase your knowledge of EBM. These include books and journals, online resources, and courses.

Books and Journals

This Concise Guide covers the basics of EBM as applied to psychiatric practice. There are a number of excellent EBM texts, each with a slightly different orientation, that provide additional information about various aspects of the EBM process. These include books by Dawes et al. (1999), Greenhalgh (2001), Guyatt and Rennie (2002a, 2002b), and Sackett et al. (2000). The texts by Dawes et al. (1999),

Greenhalgh (2001), and Guyatt and Rennie (2002a) are similar in scope to the present volume, whereas the texts of Guyatt and Rennie (2002b) and Sackett et al. (2000) provide a more in-depth coverage of topics. Although the texts are more oriented toward internists or family practitioners, they can profitably be read by anyone who wants to apply EBM to psychiatric practice.

In addition to books specifically about EBM, books about the basic sciences behind EBM (i.e., clinical epidemiology and biostatistics) may be helpful. The best starting point for learning more about clinical epidemiology is the brief clinically oriented text by Fletcher et al. (1996); Gordis (2000) has written a useful text that is slightly more detailed. Among the many biostatistics texts, the monograph by Daly and Bourke (2000) stands out for its clarity and clinical relevance.

Several journals also regularly include useful overviews of EBM concepts, including the *ACP Journal Club*, *Evidence-Based Mental Health*, and the general medical journals *BMJ* (*British Medical Journal*) and *JAMA* (*Journal of the American Medical Association*).

Internet Resources

In addition to print resources, there are a number of online resources that may be useful in learning more about various aspects of EBM. Some of the more useful sites are listed in Table 13–1.

Courses

Most medical libraries regularly offer courses about *MEDLINE* and other databases. In addition, medical librarians can be quite helpful in teaching you how to improve your search techniques.

There are also several regularly offered courses on EBM that use active small-group teaching strategies. Many of these are listed on the EBM Education Center of Excellence Web site (http://www.hsl.unc.edu/ahec/ebmcoe/pages/learning.htm). For psychiatrists, the Centre for Evidence-Based Mental Health (CEBMH) at

TABLE 13–1. **Web sites for learning more about evidence-based medicine**

Organization	Address
Centre for Evidence-Based Medicine (Oxford)	http://www.cebm.net/index.asp
Centre for Evidence-Based Medicine (Toronto)	http://www.cebm.utoronto.ca
Centre for Evidence-Based Mental Health	http://www.cebmh.com
Centre for Health Evidence	http://www.cche.net/che/home.asp
Duke University Medical Center Library	http://www.mclibrary.duke.edu/respub/guides/ebm/index.html
EBM Education Center of Excellence	http://www.hsl.unc.edu/ahec/ebmcoe/pages
Evidence-Based Medicine Resource Center	http://www.ebmny.org
NHS Critical Appraisal Skills Programme	http://www.phru.org.uk/~casp/casp.htm
Netting the Evidence	http://www.shef.ac.uk/~scharr/ir/netting
University of Oxford Cairns Library	http://www.medicine.ox.ac.uk/cairns/ebm
University of Sheffield MSc in Health Informatics	http://www.shef.ac.uk/~scharr/ir/mschi/
Users' Guides to the Medical Literature	http://ugi.usersguides.org

Oxford University offers an outstanding annual multiday course; details are available on the CEBMH Web site (http://www .cebmh.com). In addition, in recent years, 1-day courses in EBM have been offered at the American Psychiatric Association's annual meetings.

■ ACCESSING INFORMATION RESOURCES

In order to practice evidence-based psychiatry, you need access to the evidence on which to base clinical decisions. Although print resources are helpful, Internet access is highly desirable. Physicians who do not yet have Internet access either at home or at work can consult the useful book by Chan et al. (2002) for guidance.

Online Databases

There are a number of useful online databases (see Chapter 4), many of which do not require a paid subscription. Notable exceptions are *Clinical Evidence*, *Evidence-Based Mental Health*, and the *Cochrane Database of Systematic Reviews*. Readers affiliated with a medical school should check with medical librarians, because many health science libraries either subscribe to these databases through Ovid or have institutional subscriptions that allow access.

Print and Personal Digital Assistant Resources

Physicians without easy Internet access can consult two excellent print resources: *Clinical Evidence* (published semiannually) and the American Psychiatric Association (APA) practice guidelines (American Psychiatric Association 2002). In addition, *Clinical Evidence* can be downloaded from its Web site (http://www. clinicalevidence.com) to a hand-held personal digital assistant. The contents are therefore available even without Internet access.

■ OVERCOMING TIME LIMITATIONS

Patient encounters generate a variety of clinical questions, some more pressing than others. It would be difficult to go through the full 5-step EBM process for each question, so some prioritization is necessary. Welch and Lurie (2000) suggested that evidence is most worth seeking for high-risk decisions (i.e., decisions about which your patients care the most or situations that occur frequently). Added to this is the need to address specific patient questions, often generated by patients having access to the Internet and other information resources (Carter and Spink 2001; Gray 2001). As noted in Chapter 2, most psychiatrists' practices fall into a limited number of diagnostic categories. After questions related to these categories have been researched, the answers should be stored for later use.

A second strategy is to use concise preappraised information sources, as discussed above and in Chapter 4. Understandably, most clinicians prefer to use such sources rather than the full 5-step process (Mayer and Piterman 1999; McColl et al. 1998; Putnam et al. 2002). Ironically, the proliferation of preappraised sources, such as *Clinical Evidence*, secondary journals, and evidence-based guidelines, requires a strategy for efficiently utilizing them (Tables 4–3 and 4–7, Chapter 4).

If a psychiatrist has access in his or her office to the information sources described above, many questions can be answered using these preappraised resources at the time of the patient visit or shortly thereafter. If not, questions should be jotted down for later research. The services of a medical librarian or clinical informatics service (see Chapter 2) should be used if the search for evidence proves too time-consuming.

■ OVERCOMING OTHER BARRIERS

Although time, information resources, and skill are individual barriers to the practice of evidence-based psychiatry, there are also a variety of organizational barriers that limit its implementation

TABLE 13–2.	Organizational barriers to evidence-based practice

Organizational constraints
Financial resources
Staffing
Training
Equipment

Policy issues
Organization of care
Financial disincentives
Policies that promote ineffective/unproven treatments

Professional beliefs
Organizational culture
Opinion leaders
Administrators
Community standards
Pharmaceutical companies

Patient expectations
Existing beliefs
Role of media in shaping expectations

Source. Derived from Corrigan et al. 2001; Haines and Donald 2002; Marinelli-Casey et al. 2002; Oxman and Flottorp 2001; Rosenheck 2001; Torrey et al. 2001.

(Table 13–2). Organizational culture and the role of opinion leaders are two of the most important barriers (Dopson et al. 2001; Haines and Donald 2002; Rosenheck 2001).

Considerable information exists on how to change the behavior of healthcare professionals (Grimshaw et al. 2002; National Health Service Centre for Reviews and Dissemination 1999; Oxman et al. 1995), most of which suggests that traditional educational approaches are ineffective. What does seem to work, though, is "academic detailing," modeled after the visits of pharmaceutical representatives, in which one-on-one interactions are used to increase the understanding of evidence-based practices (Chilvers et al. 2002; Markey and Schattner 2001; O'Brien et al. 2002). Enlisting opinion leaders may also be helpful (Davies 1999; Dopson et al. 2001; Oxman et al. 1995). A variety of other approaches for implementing evidence-based practice in mental health organizations are presented in a recent series of articles in *Psychiatric Services* (Corrigan et al. 2001; Marinelli-Casey et al. 2002; Rosenheck 2001; Torrey et al. 2001).

■ REFERENCES

American Psychiatric Association: Practice Guidelines for the Treatment of Psychiatric Disorders: Compendium 2002. Washington, DC, American Psychiatric Association, 2002

Carter M, Spink JD: Consuming the evidence: consumers and evidence-based medicine. Med J Aust 175:316–319, 2001

Chan CH, Luo JS, Kennedy RS: Concise Guide to Computers in Clinical Psychiatry. Washington, DC, American Psychiatric Publishing, 2002

Chilvers R, Harrison G, Sipos A, et al: Evidence into practice: applications of psychological models of change in evidence-based implementation. Br J Psychiatry 181:99–101, 2002

Corrigan PW, Steiner L, McCracken SG, et al: Strategies for disseminating evidence-based practices to staff who treat people with serious mental illnesses. Psychiatr Serv 52:1598–1606, 2001

Craig JC, Irwig LM, Stockler MR: Evidence-based medicine: useful tools for decision making. Med J Aust 174:248–253, 2001

Daly LE, Bourke GJ: Interpretation and Uses of Medical Statistics, 5th Edition. Oxford, UK, Blackwell Scientific, 2000

Davies P: Introducing change, in Evidence-Based Practice: A Primer for Health Care Professionals. Edited by Dawes M, Davies P, Gray A, et al. New York, Churchill Livingstone, 1999, pp 203–218

Dawes M, Davies P, Gray A, et al. (eds): New York, Churchill Livingstone, 1999

Dopson S, Locock L, Chambers D, et al: Implementation of evidence-based medicine: evaluation of the Promoting Action on Clinical Effectiveness programme. J Health Serv Res Policy 6:23–31, 2001

Ely JW, Osheroff JA, Ebell MH, et al: Obstacles to answering doctors' questions about patient care with evidence: qualitative study. BMJ 324:710–713, 2002

Fletcher RH, Fletcher SW, Wagner EH: Clinical Epidemiology: The Essentials, 3rd Edition. Baltimore, MD, Williams & Wilkins, 1996

Geddes J, Carney S: Recent advances in evidence-based psychiatry. Can J Psychiatry 46:403–406, 2001

Gordis L: Epidemiology, 2nd Edition. Philadelphia, PA, WB Saunders, 2000

Gray JAM: Evidence-Based Healthcare: How to Make Health Policy and Management Decisions, 2nd Edition. New York, Churchill Livingstone, 2001

Greenhalgh T: How to Read a Paper: The Basics of Evidence Based Medicine, 2nd Edition. London, BMJ Books, 2001

Grimshaw J, Shirran L, Thomas R, et al: Changing provider behaviour: an overview of systematic reviews of interventions to promote implementation of research findings by healthcare professionals, in Getting Research Findings into Practice, 2nd Edition. Edited by Haines A, Donald A. London, BMJ Books, 2002, pp 29–67

Guyatt G, Rennie D (eds): Users' Guides to the Medical Literature: Essentials of Evidence-Based Clinical Practice. Chicago, IL, AMA Press, 2002a

Guyatt G, Rennie D (eds): Users' Guides to the Medical Literature: A Manual for Evidence-Based Clinical Practice. Chicago, IL, AMA Press, 2002b

Haines A, Donald A: Introduction, in Getting Research Findings into Practice, 2nd Edition. Edited by Haines A, Donald A. London, BMJ Books, 2002, pp 1–10

Marinelli-Casey P, Domier CP, Rawson RA: The gap between research and practice in substance abuse treatment. Psychiatr Serv 53:984–987, 2002

Markey P, Schattner P: Promoting evidence-based medicine in general practice: the impact of academic detailing. Fam Pract 18:364–366, 2001

Mayer J, Piterman L: The attitudes of Australian GPs to evidence-based medicine: a focus group study. Fam Pract 16:627–632, 1999

McColl A, Smith S, White P, et al: General practitioners' perceptions of the route to evidence based medicine: a questionnaire survey. BMJ 316:361–365, 1998

National Health Service Centre for Reviews and Dissemination: Getting evidence into practice. Eff Health Care 5(1):1–16, 1999

O'Brien T, Oxman AD, Davis, DA, et al: Educational outreach visits: effects on professional practice and health care outcomes, in The Cochrane Library, Issue 1. Oxford, UK, Update Software, 2002

Oxman AD, Flottorp S: An overview of strategies to promote implementation of evidence-based health care, in Evidence-Based Practice in Primary Care, 2nd Edition. Edited by Silagy C, Haines A. London, BMJ Books, 2001, pp 101–119

Oxman AD, Thomson MA, Davis DA, et al: No magic bullets: a systematic review of 102 trials of interventions to improve professional practice. CMAJ 153:1423–1431, 1995

Putnam W, Twohig PL, Burge FI, et al: A qualitative study of evidence in primary care: what the practitioners are saying. CMAJ 166:1525–1530, 2002

Rosenheck RA: Organizational process: a missing link between research and practice. Psychiatr Serv 52:1607–1612, 2001

Sackett DL, Straus SE, Richardson WS, et al: Evidence-Based Medicine: How to Practice and Teach EBM, 2nd Edition. New York, Churchill Livingstone, 2000

Torrey WC, Drake RE, Dixon L, et al: Implementing evidence-based practices for persons with severe mental illnesses. Psychiatr Serv 52:45–50, 2001

Welch HG, Lurie JD: Teaching evidence-based medicine: caveats and challenges. Acad Med 75:235–240, 2000

Young JM, Ward JE: Evidence-based medicine in general practice: beliefs and barriers among Australian GPs. J Eval Clin Pract 7:201–211, 2001

TEACHING EVIDENCE-BASED MEDICINE TO PSYCHIATRY RESIDENTS

This chapter is intended as a brief overview for residency directors and faculty who are responsible for teaching evidence-based medicine (EBM) to their residents. Other useful sources of information about teaching EBM include the works of Davies (1999), the Evidence-Based Medicine Working Group (1992), Gray (2001), Green (2000), and Sackett et al. (2000).

■ WHY TEACH EVIDENCE-BASED MEDICINE?

For over a decade, teaching medical students and residents the fundamentals of clinical epidemiology and EBM has been viewed as a way of enabling them to keep up with the medical literature and of improving clinical care (Evidence-Based Medicine Working Group 1992; Sackett et al. 1991). More recently, however, it has become a required part of residency education in the United States.

The Accreditation Council for Graduate Medical Education (ACGME) introduced general competencies for residents that are to be included in the requirements for all specialties (ACGME 2001a). Although the competencies do not use the term *evidence-based medicine*, it is clear that they require that residents become competent in the EBM process. For example, the "patient care" competency requirement of the ACGME (2001a)—that residents be able to "make informed decisions about diagnostic and therapeutic interventions based on patient information and preferences, up-to-date scientific evidence, and clinical judgment"—is remarkably similar to the model for the evidence-based clinical decisions of Haynes et al. (2002). The "practice-based learning and improvement" competency requires that residents be able to "locate, appraise, and assimilate evidence from scientific studies related to their patients' health problems," "apply knowledge of study designs and statistical methods to the appraisal of clinical studies and other information on diagnostic and therapeutic effectiveness," and "use information technology to ... access on-line medical information..." (ACGME 2001a). This encompasses steps 2–4 of the EBM model described in Chapter 2.

The most recent requirements for psychiatry residency programs (ACGME 2002) similarly require that programs teach EBM. Requirement V.A.2.b.12, for example, requires that residents have experience in critical appraisal of the literature, and requirement VI.B.1 requires that programs assess resident competence in the ACGME core skills, including practice-based learning and improvement.

■ WHAT TO TEACH

The ACGME general competencies require that psychiatry residents become competent in using the EBM process to answer questions regarding therapies and diagnostic tests. At a minimum, therefore, residents should be taught how to formulate a clinical question (Chapter 3); perform a literature search (Chapter 4); appraise clinical trials, systematic reviews, guidelines, and diagnostic tests (Chapters 5–8); and apply the results to their patients. A more complete course would include appraisal of articles on disease frequency (Chapter 9), etiology or harm (Chapter 10), and prognosis (Chapter 11).

In providing this instruction, it is important to realize that most residents are not interested in clinical epidemiology or in learning some of the more advanced EBM skills (Guyatt et al. 2000). The goal instead should be to ensure that residents are able to efficiently find answers using the preappraised information sources described in Chapter 4 (Evans 2001; Guyatt et al. 2000). There are, however, times when preappraised sources will not yield an answer or when it is necessary to discuss the evidence in more detail with a colleague or patient. Under these circumstances, it is necessary to have the kind of deeper knowledge that is covered in an advanced course (Woodcock et al. 2002). Furthermore, a deeper understanding of EBM allows clinicians to better appraise the quality of guidelines developed by others and to better understand and incorporate the results from systematic reviews into clinical practice (Doust and Silagy 2000; Laupacis 2001).

One of the more important aspects of teaching EBM to psychiatry residents is teaching the philosophy of EBM, not just the methodology. Residents often have a number of misconceptions about EBM (Bilsker and Goldner 1999; Padrino 2002). In addition to providing an overview of what EBM is and what it is not (see Chapter 1) and discussing some of the misconceptions about EBM (Straus and McAlister 2000), it may be helpful to distribute the humorous article by Isaacs and Fitzgerald (1999), in which they describe alternatives to EBM, such as *eminence-based medicine* ("experience... is worth any amount of evidence"), *vehemence-based medicine* ("substitution of volume for evidence"), and *eloquence-based medicine*. This article is also helpful to residents in coping with situations in which the opinions of their supervisors are at odds with the evidence in the literature.

■ METHODS OF TEACHING EVIDENCE-BASED MEDICINE

Individuals experienced in teaching EBM to medical students or residents favor the use of active teaching methods in small group settings (Davies 1999; Green 2000; Sackett et al. 2000). In my program, and in many others, this usually involves a combination of approaches, including seminars, journal clubs, computer lab/library sessions, and coverage during supervision or rounds.

Seminars and Small Group Sessions

Some material can best be introduced in seminars or in small group sessions. In my program, I introduce a topic (e.g., critical appraisal of clinical trials) to a small group in the form of a brief presentation and discussion. This is then followed by the critical appraisal of an article related to the topic under discussion (e.g., an article reporting the results of a randomized controlled trial). To do the appraisal, the residents are given a copy of the article and a worksheet that incorporates the appropriate critical appraisal guidelines. After the residents have all completed the worksheet, individual items on it are discussed. Although such sessions are useful for introducing a topic or method, they do not provide sufficient practice for the residents to become proficient; for this, other approaches are more useful.

Computer Lab and Library Sessions

The best way to become familiar with the various databases and how to use them is through hands-on practice, not by reading about them or through a lecture. Most medical schools have computer labs or library classrooms equipped with computers that can be used for demonstrations and hands-on practice in a group setting. Most medical libraries offer classes on searching *MEDLINE* and other databases, and librarians will often customize courses for the needs of particular users. For example, our residents receive instruction in searching the Ovid *Evidence-Based Medicine Reviews* database, which includes the Cochrane systematic reviews and *DARE*.

Evidence-Based Journal Clubs

Journal clubs, a staple of residency education programs, are the most common sites for teaching critical appraisal skills (Green 1999, 2000). Sackett et al. (2000) have described a novel approach to journal clubs, the evidence-based journal club, as a method for teaching the EBM process.

In an evidence-based journal club, the starting point is a clinical question suggested by one of the residents, preferably one that is based on an actual patient care issue. The group agrees on the 4-part PICO question (a question that uses the mnemonic aid "patient/problem, intervention, comparison, and outcome"), and a resident is assigned to conduct a literature search to find the best evidence to answer the question. The resident assigned to the task tries to find the evidence that is highest in the hierarchy (Table 4–2, Chapter 4). At the next journal club meeting, the resident distributes the article that was found, and the group as a whole uses a critical appraisal worksheet to evaluate the article. The question, search process, results, and applicability are then discussed.

The evidence-based journal club format has become popular in psychiatry training programs in the United Kingdom (Dhar 2001; Walker 2001; Warner and King 1997); however, such a format is uncommon in psychiatry residency programs in the United States (G.E. Gray, unpublished data, 2001).

Rounds and Supervision

It is generally recommended that EBM not be taught in isolation, but instead be incorporated in other clinical teaching activities (Dobbie et al. 2000; Green 1999, 2000; Sackett et al. 2000). In some institutions, this can be done through real-time literature searches during rounds or supervision, but online database access is still the exception in most hospital settings (Green 2000). Sackett et al. (2000) and the Evidence-Based Medicine Working Group (1992), for example, describe settings in which online searches can be conducted during rounds. I have residents come to my office for individual supervision, and in that setting clinical questions can be answered on the spot, on the basis of the online retrieval of appropriate evidence.

Educational Prescriptions

In many cases, lack of time or Internet access precludes real-time literature searches. Under these circumstances, the resident can be assigned the task of conducting the search and bringing back the evidence for the next session. *Educational prescriptions* can be used to formally assign the task (Sackett et al. 2000). Such prescriptions specify the problem, the question, and who is responsible for answering it; in addition, a deadline is given, as is a reminder to all parties of the steps involved (Centre for Evidence-Based Medicine n.d., 2000).

■ ONLINE TEACHING RESOURCES

A variety of Web sites provide useful information (such as curriculum guides and online syllabi) for the teaching of EBM (Table 14–1).

Critical Appraisal Worksheets

Worksheets for critically appraising various types of articles can be downloaded from the Web sites of the Centre for Evidence-Based Medicine and the Centre for Evidence-Based Mental Health (Table 14–1). Such worksheets parallel the critical appraisal guidelines given in this Concise Guide and are quite helpful both in teaching critical appraisal skills and in running journal clubs.

Educational Prescription Forms

Educational prescription forms can be downloaded from the Web sites of the Centre for Evidence-Based Medicine in Toronto (http://www.cebm.utoronto.ca/practise/formulate/eduprescript.htm) or Oxford (http://www.cebm.net/index.asp).

Personal Digital Assistant Resources

The use of personal digital assistants (PDAs) by medical students and residents, including by those in psychiatry training programs, is becoming increasingly popular (Cameron 2002; Criswell and Parchman 2002; Luo et al. 2002; Stoddard 2001). A variety of

TABLE 14–1. **Useful sites for teachers of evidence-based medicine**

Organization	Address
Centre for Evidence-Based Medicine (Oxford)	http://www.cebm.net/index.asp
Centre for Evidence-Based Medicine (Toronto)	http://www.cebm.utoronto.ca/teach/
Centre for Evidence-Based Mental Health	http://www.cebmh.com
EBM Education Center of Excellence	http://www.hsl.unc.edu/ahec/ebmcoe/pages
Evidence-Based Medicine Resource Center	http://www.ebmny.org/teach.html

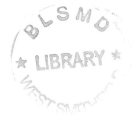

resources to support the learning of EBM are now available for PDAs using the Palm operating system (Table 14–2).

■ EVALUATING EVIDENCE-BASED MEDICINE SKILLS

Most evaluations of EBM have focused on critical appraisal skills of knowledge of EBM terminology and concepts, generally using multiple-choice exams (Green 1999, 2000; Hatala and Guyatt 2002). Such approaches suffer from many criticisms, including the lack of validation of instruments and failure to assess the entire EBM process.

One promising approach for appraising a broader range of EBM skills is that of Smith et al. (2000), who developed a written test that focuses on four different skills: formulation of questions, literature searches, quantitative understanding, and appraisal of study quality and clinical relevance. Other authors have suggested the use of objective structured clinical exam–type stations to assess specific skills (Dobbie et al. 2000).

Evaluating whether residents are applying EBM skills in their day-to-day practices is as yet an unmet need. Such assessments have generally relied on self-reports, which may not be accurate (Green 1999, 2000). For example, Cabell et al. (2001) found that resident self-reports overestimate the actual use of online databases.

The ACGME Outcome Project (ACGME 2001b) has suggested a number of approaches to assessing practice-based learning and improvement competency. Included are self-administered diaries, portfolios, and instruments to assess opinions about EBM and information technology; and knowledge of EBM concepts and critical appraisal skills. The test of Smith et al. (2000), described earlier in this section, is included in the examples.

In my psychiatry residency program, competency is assessed through residents' preparation of a portfolio of critically appraised topics (CATs) generated in the evidence-based journal club. As described in Chapter 2 of this volume, CATs are short summaries of

TABLE 14–2. **Evidence-based medicine resources for personal digital assistants**

Clinical Evidence (http://www.clinicalevidence.com)

Can download portions or entire sections, either summaries or full text

EBM Calculator (http://www.cebm.utoronto.ca/palm/ebmcalc)

For randomized controlled trials, calculates relative risk reduction, absolute risk reduction, number needed to treat, and confidence intervals

For diagnostic test, calculates sensitivity, specificity, positive and negative predictive values, and likelihood ratios

For epidemiologic studies, calculates relative risk, odds ratio, etc.

EBM Tables (http://www.cebm.utoronto.ca/palm/nnt)

Number needed to treat tables include numbers need to treat for various therapies

Likelihood ratio tables include LR+ and LR– for various diagnostic tests

SnNout/SpPin tables include sensitivities and specificities of various diagnostic tests

EBM Tool Kit (http://www.mclibrary.duke.edu/respub/pdaformat/ebm.html)

Evidence-based medicine glossary

Well-built clinical question

Ovid *MEDLINE* guide

Critical appraisal checklists

Statistical/epidemiologic concepts (e.g., number needed to treat, sensitivity, LR+, etc.)

Search filters

A Student's Guide to the Medical Literature (http://denison.uchsc.edu/SG/PDA.html)

Framing the question

Information resources

Search strategies

Critical appraisal checklists

Glossary of statistical terms

Note. LR+=likelihood ratio of a positive test; LR–=likelihood ratio of a negative test; SnNout=**Sen**sitive test, **N**egative result, rules **out** disease; SpPin=**Sp**ecific test, **P**ositive test, rules **in** disease.

answers to clinical questions. Preparation of a CAT involves formulating a question, searching for an answer, and appraising the evidence. A sample CAT format is given in Table 14–3, and further details can be found in the works of Badenoch (2002), Badenoch and Heneghan (2002), and Sackett et al. (2000).

■ RESIDENT VIEWS OF EVIDENCE-BASED MEDICINE

Psychiatry residents often have some exposure to EBM as medical students, although this is not necessarily true for international medical graduates. Residents often have some ambivalence toward EBM, wondering if it ignores the humanistic side of psychiatric practice (Bilsker and Goldner 1999). However, as they develop a better understanding of EBM and the roles of clinical judgment and patient preference, coming to realize that EBM and patient-centered care are complementary, such concerns generally lessen (Bilsker and Goldner 1999; Hope 2002).

Some residents are intimidated by the quantitative emphasis of EBM (Bilsker and Goldner 1999). This can generally be overcome by setting realistic goals and by remembering that the focus should be on preparing users of evidence, not researchers (Guyatt et al. 2000; Sackett et al. 2000).

Some of the other barriers to the practice of EBM that residents face, including lack of time and access to information resources, are similar to those encountered by practicing physicians (Cabell et al. 2001). As discussed in Chapter 13, these barriers can often be overcome by making preappraised information resources available (Evans 2001; Geddes and Carney 2001; Guyatt et al. 2000).

An added barrier, however, may be the negative opinions of some faculty members (Ball 1999; Evidence-Based Medicine Working Group 1992). Faculty development efforts may be needed to address the negative opinions (Bilsker and Goldner 1999; Evidence-Based Medicine Working Group 1992; Neale et al. 1999), al-

TABLE 14–3. Outline for a critically appraised topic (CAT)

Title of the CAT	A declarative statement that provides the answer to your clinical question
Clinical bottom line	One or two sentences that briefly describe the results of the article
Citation	Reference to the article that was appraised
Clinical question	A 4-part PICO question ("patient/problem, intervention, comparison, and outcome") format
Search terms used and database(s) searched	A list documenting the search
The study	A brief description of the study design, number of subjects, subject selection criteria, outcome measures, etc.
The results	Results should be presented in a table. Use dichotomous outcome measures and calculate number needed to treat and confidence intervals
Comments	Any additional information of note
Appraised by	Name of person preparing the CAT
Appraisal date	Useful information as an indication of when an updated search may be necessary

Source. Based on Badenoch 2002; Badenoch and Heneghan 2002; Sackett et al. 2000.

though some residents are able to educate their supervisors about the concepts (Ball 1999). In my program, residents report that they have found the Isaacs and Fitzgerald (1999) article useful for putting their supervisors' criticisms of EBM in perspective.

Finally, it is important to emphasize that many residents find the practice of EBM to be empowering (Ball 1998; Padrino 2002). As Padrino (2002) said, "I feel more confident in my medical decisions when I can say 'the data show this' or 'the data show that.' Even when I have to say 'there are no data for this,' I feel my decision is more valid" (p. 13). Being able to incorporate the best evidence from the research literature into patient care decisions is what EBM is all about, and residents are quite capable of learning how to use evidence to improve their clinical decision making.

■ REFERENCES

Accreditation Council for Graduate Medical Education: General competencies [ACGME Outcome Project Web site]. 2001a. Available at: http://www.acgme.org/outcome/comp/compFull.asp. Accessed October 22, 2002

Accreditation Council for Graduate Medical Education: Practice-based learning and improvement: assessment approaches [ACGME Outcome Project Web site]. 2001b. Available at: http://www.acgme.org/outcome/assess/PBLI_Index.asp. Accessed October 29, 2002

Accreditation Council for Graduate Medical Education: Program requirements for residency training in psychiatry [ACGME Web site]. 2002. Available at: http://www.acgme.org/req/400pr101.asp. Accessed October 22, 2002

Badenoch D: What is a CAT? [Centre for Evidence-Based Medicine Web site]. May 31, 2002. Available at: http://www.cebm.net/cat_about.asp. Accessed June 28, 2003

Badenoch D, Heneghan C: Evidence-Based Medicine Toolkit. London, BMJ Books, 2002

Ball C: Evidence-based medicine on the wards: report from an evidence-based minion. Evidence-Based Medicine 3:101–103, 1999

Bilsker D, Goldner EM: Teaching evidence-based practice in mental health. Evid Based Ment Health 2:68–69, 1999

Cabell CH, Schardt C, Sanders L, et al: Resident utilization of information technology: a randomized trial of clinical question formation. J Gen Intern Med 16:838–844, 2001

Cameron S: Handheld computers in medicine. Can Fam Physician 48:111–112, 2002

Centre for Evidence-Based Medicine: Educational prescriptions [Centre for Evidence-Based Medicine Web site]. n.d. Available at: http://www.cebm.net/eduscrip.asp. Accessed June 28, 2003

Centre for Evidence-Based Medicine: What is an educational prescription? [Centre for Evidence-Based Medicine Web site]. 2000. Available at: http://www.cebm.utoronto.ca/practise/formulate/eduprescript.htm. Accessed October 28, 2002

Criswell DF, Parchman ML: Handheld computer use in U.S. family practice residency programs. J Am Med Inform Assoc 9:80–86, 2002

Davies P: Teaching evidence-based health care, in Evidence-Based Practice: A Primer for Health Care Professionals. Edited by Dawes M, Davies P, Gray A, et al. New York, Churchill Livingstone, 1999, pp 223–242

Dhar R: Evidence-based journal clubs and the critical review paper: candidate's perspective. Psychiatr Bull 25:67–68, 2001

Dobbie AE, Schneider ED, Anderson AD, et al: What evidence supports teaching evidence-based medicine? Acad Med 75:1184–1185, 2000

Doust JA, Silagy CA: Applying the results of a systematic review in general practice. Med J Aust 172:153–156, 2000

Evans M: Creating knowledge management skills in primary care residents: a description of a new pathway to evidence-based practice. ACP J Club 135:A11–A12, 2001

Evidence-Based Medicine Working Group: Evidence-based medicine: a new approach to teaching the practice of medicine. JAMA 268:2420–2425, 1992

Geddes J, Carney S: Recent advances in evidence-based psychiatry. Can J Psychiatry 46:403–406, 2001

Gray JAM: Evidence-Based Healthcare: How to Make Health Policy and Management Decisions, 2nd Edition. New York, Churchill Livingstone, 2001

Green ML: Graduate medical education training in clinical epidemiology, critical appraisal, and evidence-based medicine: a critical review of curricula. Acad Med 74:686–694, 1999

Green ML: Evidence-based medicine training in graduate medical education: past, present, and future. J Eval Clin Pract 6:121–138, 2000

Guyatt GH, Meade MO, Jaeschke RZ, et al: Practitioners of evidence-based care. BMJ 320:954–955, 2000

Hatala R, Guyatt G: Evaluating the teaching of evidence-based medicine. JAMA 288:1110–1112, 2002

Haynes RB, Devereaux PJ, Guyatt GH: Physicians' and patients' choices in evidence based practice. BMJ 324:1350, 2002

Hope T: Evidence-based patient choice and psychiatry. Evid Based Ment Health 5:100–101, 2002

Isaacs D, Fitzgerald D: Seven alternatives to evidence based medicine. BMJ 319:1618, 1999

Laupacis A: The future of evidence-based medicine. Can J Clin Pharmacol 8 (suppl A):6A–9A, 2001

Luo J, Hales RE, Servis M, et al: Use of personal digital assistants in consultation psychiatry. Psychiatr Serv 53:271–272; 279, 2002

Neale V, Roth LM, Schwartz KL: Faculty development using evidence-based medicine as an organizing curricular theme. Acad Med 74:611, 1999

Padrino S: Evidence-based psychiatry: fad or fundamental? Psychiatr News 37(16):13, 2002

Sackett DL, Haynes RB, Guyatt GH, et al: Clinical Epidemiology: A Basic Science for Clinical Medicine, 2nd Edition. Boston, MA, Little, Brown, 1991

Sackett DL, Strauss SE, Richardson WS, et al: Evidence-Based Medicine: How to Practice and Teach EBM, 2nd Edition. New York, Churchill Livingstone, 2000

Smith CA, Ganschow PS, Reilly BM: Teaching residents evidence-based medicine skills: a controlled trial of effectiveness and assessment of durability. J Gen Intern Med 15:710–715, 2000

Stoddard M: PDA initiatives in health care libraries [Arizona Health Sciences Library Web site]. November 2001. Available at: http://educ.ahsl.arizona.edu/pda/lib.htm. Accessed October 28, 2002

Straus SE, McAlister FA: Evidence-based medicine: a commentary on common criticisms. CMAJ 163:837–841, 2000

Walker N: Evidence-based journal clubs and the critical review paper. Psychiatr Bull 25:237, 2001

Warner JP, King M: Evidence-based medicine and the journal club: a cross-sectional survey of participants' views. Psychiatr Bull 21:532–534, 1997

Woodcock JD, Greenley S, Barton S: Doctors' knowledge about evidence-based medicine terminology. BMJ 324:929–930, 2002

Appendix A

GLOSSARY

absolute risk increase (ARI)   Difference between experimental event rate (EER) and control event rate (CER) when a treatment increases the risk of a negative outcome.

absolute risk reduction (ARR)   Difference between control event rate (CER) and experimental event rate (EER) when a treatment decreases the risk of a negative outcome.

allocation concealment   Refers to whether the person making the allocation of a patient to either the experimental or control treatment in a randomized controlled trial is aware of the group to which the next patient will be assigned.

alpha (α)   Probability of a type I error (i.e., falsely concluding that there is a difference between the experimental and control groups when such a difference is the result of chance alone).

attributable risk   Difference in incidence rates between exposed and nonexposed cohorts; also known as *risk difference* (RD).

beta (β)   Probability of a type II error (i.e., falsely concluding that there is no difference between the experimental and control groups when such a difference in fact exists).

bias   Systematic deviation of the results from the truth.

blinded or blind   Refers to whether patients, clinicians, raters, and data analysts are aware of which treatment a patient in a trial is receiving. Although terms like *single blind*, *double blind*, or *triple blind* are sometimes used, there is no consistent meaning to them, and it is better to specify which participants have been blinded.

case report   Description of a single case.

case series   Description of a series of cases.

case-control study   Observational study in which exposure to a suspected risk factor is assessed in cases with the disease and in control subjects without the disease.

cohort   A group of persons followed over time.

cohort study   An observational study in which a cohort is followed over time and the number of cases of disease (or another outcome measure) is assessed. Typically, the cohort is divided into those who are exposed to a potential risk factor and those who are not exposed, and the difference or ratio of incidence rates is computed.

cointervention   Intervention other than the treatment under study that is applied differentially to the control and experimental groups.

confidence interval (CI)   Range of values in which the true value most likely lies.

confounding variable   Variable related to the outcome, which differs in frequency between the experimental (or exposed) and control (or nonexposed) groups. Confounding variables, not the variable under study, may be responsible for observed differences in the groups.

control event rate (CER)   Rate of events in the control (nonexposed or nonexperimental) group. Typically expressed in terms of negative events.

cross-product ratio   Odds ratio.

cross-sectional survey   Observational study design in which exposures and outcomes are determined at the same point in time.

dichotomous outcome   Outcome that can take only two values (e.g., dead or alive).

effect size   Measure of the difference in outcomes between the control and experimental groups.

experimental event rate (EER)   Rate of events in the experimental (exposed) group. Typically expressed in terms of negative events.

Hawthorne effect   Performance improves when subjects know they are being studied.

inception cohort   Group of people assembled at a common point, early in the course of their illnesses.

incidence   Number of new cases of disease in a population in a given period of time.

intention-to-treat analysis   Statistical analysis that includes all patients assigned to a treatment group, regardless of whether they completed study.

Kaplan-Meier curve   Survival curve.

likelihood ratio (LR)   Relative likelihood of test results in those with disease, compared with those without disease.

meta-analysis   Statistical technique that pools results from more than one study to yield a summary result.

negative predictive value (NPV)   Proportion of negative test results that are true negatives.

number needed to harm (NNH)   Number of patients that must be treated with an experimental therapy to produce one additional bad outcome that would not have occurred on the control therapy. Inverse of *absolute risk increase.*

number needed to treat (NNT)   Number of patients that must be treated with an experimental therapy to prevent one bad outcome that would have occurred on the control therapy. Inverse of *absolute risk reduction.*

odds   Ratio of the probability of an event occurring to the probability of an event not occurring.

odds ratio (OR)   Ratio of odds of event in exposed group to odds of event in nonexposed group. In a case-control study, ratio of odds of exposure in cases to odds of exposure in control subjects; also known as *cross-product ratio.*

patient expected event rate   Expected risk of negative outcomes in patient if control treatment is administered.

positive predictive value (PPV)   Proportion of positive test results that are true positives.

posttest odds   Odds of disease in patient after results of test are known.

posttest probability   Probability of disease in patient after results of test are known.

pretest odds   Odds of disease in patient before results of test are known.

pretest probability   Probability of disease in patient before results of test are known.

prevalence   Proportion of persons in a population with disease of interest.

randomization   Allocation of subjects to groups by chance.

randomized controlled trial (RCT)   Clinical trial in which patients are randomly allocated to control or experimental treatment groups.

receiver operating characteristic curve (ROC)   Plot of false positive rate (1–specificity) versus true positive rate (sensitivity).

relative risk (RR)   In a cohort study, ratio of incidence of disease in exposed group to incidence in nonexposed group. In a randomized controlled trial, ratio of rate of negative events in experimental group (EER) to rate in control group (CER).

relative risk reduction (RRR)   In an randomized controlled trial, proportion of risk of negative outcome reduced by the experimental therapy. Calculated as 1–relative risk (RR).

reliability   Degree to which results are reproducible.

risk difference (RD)   Difference in incidence rates between exposed and nonexposed cohorts.

risk factor   Patient characteristic that increases risk of disease.

risk ratio   Relative risk.

sensitivity   Proportion of persons with a disease who are correctly identified by a diagnostic test.

specificity   Proportion of persons without a disease who are correctly identified by a diagnostic test.

survival analysis   Method of analyzing time-to-event data.

survival curve   Graphical display of proportion of individuals who have not had event occur, plotted over time.

systematic review   Literature review that involves comprehensive search for relevant articles, followed by critical appraisal and summarizing of articles that meet quality criteria.

type I error   Falsely concluding that there is a difference between experimental and control groups when such a difference is the result of chance alone.

type II error   Falsely concluding that there is no difference between experimental and control groups when such a difference in fact exists.

validity   Degree to which results of a study are unbiased.

Appendix B

STATISTICAL FORMULAS AND TABLES

B–1: Confidence intervals for number needed to treat and number needed to harm

B–2: Calculating patient-specific number needed to treat and number needed to harm estimates

B–3: Calculating the likelihood of being helped versus harmed by a therapy

B–4: Calculating number needed to treat and number needed to harm from the odds ratio

B–5: Interpreting standardized effect size

■ BIBLIOGRAPHY

Freemantle N, Geddes J: Understanding and interpreting systematic reviews and meta-analyses, II: meta-analyses. Evid Based Ment Health 1:102–104, 1998

Leung R: Appendix: calculations, in Users' Guides to the Medical Literature: A Manual for Evidence-Based Clinical Practice. Edited by Guyatt GH, Rennie D. Chicago, IL, AMA Press, 2002, pp 659–664

Sackett DL, Straus SE, Richardson WS, et al: Evidence-Based Medicine: How to Practice and Teach EBM, 2nd Edition. New York, Churchill Livingstone, 2000

TABLE B–1.   **Confidence intervals (CIs) for number needed to treat and number needed to harm**

	Experimental treatment	Control treatment
Bad outcome	A	B
Good outcome	C	D
Total	n_1	n_2

Control event rate (CER) = B/n_2
Experimental event rate (EER) = A/n_1

If treatment leads to fewer bad outcomes:

Absolute risk reduction (ARR) = CER − EER
Number needed to treat (NNT) = 1/ARR
Standard error of ARR (SE_{ARR}) = $\{[(CER)(1-CER)/n_2]+[(EER)(1-EER)/n_1]\}^{1/2}$
Upper limit of 95% CI for ARR (U_{ARR}) = ARR + 1.96 SE_{ARR}
Lower limit of 95% CI for ARR (L_{ARR}) = ARR − 1.96 SE_{ARR}
Upper limit of 95% CI for NNT (U_{NNT}) = $1/L_{ARR}$
Lower limit of 95% CI for NNT (L_{NNT}) = $1/U_{ARR}$

If treatment leads to more bad outcomes:

Absolute risk increase (ARI) = EER − CER
Number needed to harm (NNH) = 1/ARI
Standard error of ARI (SE_{ARI}) = $\{[(CER)(1-CER)/n_2]+[(EER)(1-EER)/n_1]\}^{1/2}$
Upper limit of 95% CI for ARR (U_{ARI}) = ARI + 1.96 SE_{ARI}
Lower limit of 95% CI for ARR (L_{ARI}) = ARR − 1.96 SE_{ARI}
Upper limit of 95% CI for NNH (U_{NNH}) = $1/L_{ARI}$
Lower limit of 95% CI for NNH (L_{NNH}) = $1/U_{AR}$

TABLE B–2. **Calculating patient-specific number needed to treat and number needed to harm estimates**

	Experimental treatment	Control treatment
Bad outcome	A	B
Good outcome	C	D
Total	n_1	n_2

Control event rate (CER)=B/n_2
Experimental event rate (EER)=A/n_1
Relative risk (RR)= EER/CER
Patient's expected event rate (PEER)=estimate of patient's risk of bad outcome on control treatment

If treatment leads to fewer bad outcomes:

Relative risk reduction (RRR)=$1-$RR
Patient's expected absolute risk reduction (PARR)=PEER$\times$RRR
Patient-specific number needed to treat (PNNT)=$1/$PARR

If treatment leads to more bad outcomes:

Relative risk increase (RRI)=RR-1
Patient's absolute risk increase (PARI)=PEER$\times$RRI
Patient-specific number needed to harm (PNNH)=$1/$PARI

TABLE B–3.   **Calculating the likelihood of being helped versus harmed by a therapy**

Step 1

Calculate the patient-specific number needed to treat (PNNT) for the desired therapeutic effect and the patient-specific number needed to harm (PNNH) for the side effect of concern (Table B-2).

Step 2

Determine the patient's relative preference (RP) for the desired effect versus the side effect. For example, if a patient feels that it is twice as bad to gain 10 kg as it is to relapse, RP=1/2.

Step 3

Calculate the likelihood of being helped or harmed (LHH), using this formula:

$$\text{LHH} = \text{PNNH}/(\text{PNNT} \times \text{RP})$$

The LHH is the relative likelihood of being helped versus harmed by a therapy, taking into account the patient's individualized risks and values.

TABLE B–4.   **Calculating number needed to treat and number needed to harm from the odds ratio**

If treatment leads to fewer bad outcomes:

$$\text{NNT} = \frac{1 - (\text{CER})(1 - \text{OR})}{(\text{CER})(1 - \text{CER})(1 - \text{OR})}$$

If treatment leads to more bad outcomes:

$$\text{NNH} = \frac{1 + (\text{CER})(1 - \text{OR})}{(\text{CER})(1 - \text{CER})(1 - \text{OR})}$$

Note.   CER=estimated control event rate; NNT=number needed to treat; NNH=number needed to harm; OR=odds ratio.

TABLE B–5.	**Interpreting standardized effect size**

Standardized effect size (d) is a measure of the degree of overlap between experimental and control groups when there is a continuous outcome measure. To interpret d, use the chart below.

$d > 0$: The average (mean) response in the experimental group is greater than this percentage of responses in the control group.

$d < 0$: The average (mean) response in the experimental group is less than this percentage of responses in the control group.

Standardized effect size (d)	Percentile
0	50
0.2	58
0.4	66
0.6	73
0.8	79
1.0	84
1.2	88
1.4	92
1.6	95
1.8	96
2.0	98
2.3	99

INDEX

*Page numbers in **boldface** type refer to tables or figures.*